Contents

MW00928570

INTRODUCTION

7 games all. Fifth set. Final round of qualifying at Wimbledon. Ever since I can remember I have dreamed of this moment, dreamed of playing at the most prestigious tournament of them all.

It's been a long journey at times. It's been an improbable journey at times. Finally, it has been a miraculous journey.

Just two years before this moment, age 18, I got some bad news. It came in the form of a fairly nonchalant sentence. I had been having some knee pain and had been trying to sort it out with the Association of Tennis Professionals doctors, but I was not getting better. In fact, I was getting worse. A lot worse. Then, a loud POP changing direction left me feeling like I had broken glass shards loosely hanging out in my knee.

"Mr. Bower, I don't want to leave you without options, but we are going to need to take approximately one third of your Patella tendon out."

The big thick tendon right under your knee cap.

"Ok cool. Let's do this. How long is the recovery time?"

"Well. Here is the thing. We are going to cut out one third of what is probably the most important tendon for human movement, with the exception of maybe the Achilles. This is going to leave you with one strand on the left side and one strand on the right side. And nothing in the middle."

Ok, Let's roll this bad boy out! I am excited. The pain has been driving me nuts, and I can't wait to get back on track!"

"Mr. Bower. I guess what I am trying to say in a delicate way is this. If your body could not stand up to the rigors of being a professional athlete with all the body parts intact, once we partially remove the patella tendon, the risks will be just too great, and if you re-injure the area after this, then your next problem is not going to be about professional tennis, it's going to be about walking. We do not believe you will be playing professional tennis again."

It's 7 all. Fifth set. 2 Years after that diagnosis, and surgery. I am a walking miracle at this point. I know that my chances of reaching really great heights are diminished, but here I am. In contention to play in the greatest tournament of them all.

What has happened in the past and what might happen in the future fades to black, as if time is being compressed by a divine piston, distilled to just this moment. Right here. Right now. I try to run around the second serve and hit my forehand, my weapon. My legs are jelly, I am tired, I am so nervous it's hard to breathe. I hit the ball on the frame and it ends up somewhere in orbit next to the Hubble space telescope. Not good.

By some intervention of the gods of tennis, I get another break-point. I think the same thing- try to find the weapon-the forehand. Go for it. I am pretty sure that second attempt ended up as one of the first man-made objects to enter interstellar space, alongside Nasa's Voyager 1. Attempt 2. Chance to reach a dream. Gone.

A double fault sets up my third break-point. I know I have to do something about myself. I am so nervous, so anxious, so tight and so stressed, that it is impossible to approach this opportunity with any degree of rational planning. Fly by the seat of your pants, reactive, hope it kinda-just-works-out has never been a successful planning tool for anyone, and I don't want to have to remember my greatest tennis opportunity as one where I went tennis-blind, overcome by every emotion in the dictionary, my mind astral-planing while my poor body was left to do the work, unaided.

I look over at the ball kid. Can I have that ball? I take the ball and roll it along the ground. The ball kid starts chasing it. I tell them no, let me get it. I NEED to get it. As I start walking to get the ball, I have about 20 seconds to have a conversation with myself. 20 seconds to sort myself out. To solve a tangled web of emotional wires, malfunctioning to a spectacular degree. Inside my head looks like all the little scientists in their white lab coats running around panicked as the nuclear reactor enters meltdown, "DEFCON 1-DEFCON 1".

I ask myself what I want. I want to play a point that's reasonable and gives me a chance to win.

Based on how tired and nervous we both are, maybe just blocking the return back and making him play will create an opportunity. Ok, let's do that.

The minute I formulated a plan, my mind shifted away from the panic state and focused on the plan instead. It was a much better feeling.

I blocked the return. He missed. I served out the match. I had just qualified for the greatest tournament in the world.

WIMBLEDON BABY!!

I remember walking up Wimbledon hill the next morning. Those giant Bronze gates. They seem foreboding. Like a bouncer at a nightclub and you mumbling something about this being your only 2 days in town and it would be really special if he let you in for a few minutes. The bouncer simply smiles and says, "You are not on the list, sir."

A row of people 4 deep and a mile long trying to get in. I look down and felt my players badge. I showed it to the gatekeeper, and those huge bronze barriers simply gave way. I was in! (To be fair, I am relatively confident that I should be credited for inventing the selfie that day, and we won't mention official reprimand from the All England Club: "Please don't hang on the statue of Rod Laver, Sir")

This book is designed as a step by step guide to exploring your potential. It's designed as a chance to start dreaming again, and a chance to go after some of your bigger ambitions.

We all have the potential to achieve something incredible. We all have the power to make those things that are important to us come into reality. What we need to know is the HOW?

Mental toughness is your ultimate weapon. It will be there for you in your darkest times, and it will provide you with the energy and resources to keep going.

This book is dedicated to helping people build themselves from the inside out. It is designed to be a tool to do the introspection, find out strengths and weaknesses, formulate action plans and start building forward momentum. It is about reimagining your values, tethering your ship to positivity and to growth. It is about self-mastery.

It is about your life as a work of art, and you the artist digging in, getting inspired and drawing on experience to create a masterpiece. It is about redefining success and chasing improvement in all areas of your life.

It is about realizing that the world wants you at your best, it wants to see your unique perspective and brilliant ideas.

What can we do to make the idea of being mentally tough, sexy? You know, Steve Jobs style. Steve Jobs, he not only saved Apple at the verge of bankruptcy in the late 90's, he launched the "Think different" advertising campaign which gave birth to the iPod, iPhone, and iPad. Jobs made sizzling, to drool over products that worked beautifully. My vision is for you to reengineer your strategies, reimagine your future, remake your belief structures and reignite your passion.

Personally, I don't want to have to go to Dubai to see the most beautiful and modern buildings on earth. I want to see them here, in America. You can't tell me we shouldn't have solved solar power by now. You can't tell me we shouldn't have solved hydroponic farming in the poor areas of the world. You can't tell me we shouldn't be nearing the end of oil usage and moving towards more abundant and less damaging fuel sources. You can't tell me that 40% of the world should still be living in poverty! We have to get on that! The world has a million unanswered questions, and it's up to us to find answers.

Perhaps, everything can be summed up by an old favorite,

O Me! O Life!

BY WALT WHITMAN

Oh me! Oh life! Of the questions of these recurring,

Of the endless trains of the faithless, of cities filled with the foolish,

Of myself forever reproaching myself,

(for who more foolish than I, and who more faithless?)

Of eyes that vainly crave the light, of the objects mean,

of the struggle ever renewed,

Of the poor results of all,

of the plodding and sordid crowds I see around me,

Of the empty and useless years of the rest, with the rest me intertwined,

The question, O me! so sad, recurring—

What good amid these, O me, O life?

Answer.

That you are here—that life exists and identity,

That the powerful play goes on, and you may contribute a verse.

Well Walt, I reckon it is time to add a verse.

CHAPTER 1: THE 9 CORE INTERNALS

Gun Powder.
Coca-Cola.
Cement.
Penicillin.
Recipes. Ingredients. Combinations and ratios. Game Changers.

Wallpaper cleaner.
This is going to take a little explaining, isn't it?

Allow me to elaborate. Way back in the day, people used to heat their homes predominantly by burning coal or wood in the fireplace. Way back in that same day, people used all kinds of fantastic derivatives of brown yellow and green kaleidoscope patterns to decorate their walls, in the form of wallpaper. Two problems sprung up. Burning things left a sooty residue all over the wallpaper, and paper by its very nature could not be cleaned by water. Which leads us to the star of our little story, Kutol. A company that made a white, doughy, wallpaper cleaner that was perfectly up to the task.

With the introduction of oil and gas fireplaces, the soot problem began to disappear, and with it, Kutol's future and profits. Enter Kay Zufall. While searching for some cheap materials for the kids to play with for Christmas decorations, she stumbled upon a Martha Stewart type article suggesting wallpaper cleaner was the perfect go-to for a cheap toy that kids could play with.

Knowing that her brother in laws company was knee deep in the red, she bought a sizeable amount of their product to see if it the article was right. The kids loved it and played for hours.

Joe McVicker (CEO of soon to be obsolete Kutol) agreed to take the soap out and add some coloring to his brand new, kid friendly product, and proposed naming it "Kutol's Rainbow Modeling Compound"

After a couple of slaps, some sarcasm and a serious questioning of his branding acumen, Kay told Joe that this name simply wouldn't do. She set about coming up with a better one, and the now legendary "Play-Doh" was born.

From wallpaper cleaner to children's toy. Ingredients. Recipes. Removing one ingredient and adding another. Unlocking a purpose no one could have seen or imagined.

That's what this chapter is all about.

We are all built from a similar emotional tool kit. We all have access to similar ingredients. Blending, adding, removing, and tinkering with how we put these ingredients together is our great puzzle, our great work of art, and the pathway to opening doors to expression of our talents that we don't even know exist yet.

Of course, just like Kutol, we often plod along doing what we know how to do and blending the ingredients in the same-old-way for years, only mixing up the recipe when we are absolutely forced to.

Had it not been for the pending bankruptcy, who knows if Play-Doh would ever have been

For however many things have a plurality of parts and are not merely a complete aggregate, but instead some kind of a whole beyond its parts...

Aristotle

You think about the difference in chromosomes between an ape and a man, and that 1% difference sure counts for a lot. What if just a couple of small changes in your own decision making, habits and choices could unlock a 1% difference that made that same kind of difference for you as it did for that ape?

If you plan to get something meaningful out of your lifetime, you are going to need to direct yourself and your energy towards the ideas you want to manifest into reality. You will want to actively seek self-mastery, and you will want to update yourself consistently as you evolve and grow.

Your tools of trade here in this lifetime are this remarkably complex piece of biological machinery called the human body and an emotional center that can, when properly trained and directed, tame some of the most extravagant ideas in the universe.

There is now ample evidence that success and the internal characteristics that facilitate success are not born characteristics. Enough people have pulled themselves up out of the gutter, have risen to conquer overwhelming odds for us to know, beyond a shadow of a doubt, that internal character traits and an emotional core that facilitates success are plastic enough, changeable enough, that they can be learned and mastered by anyone.

Our lives, and ultimately, our destiny will be determined by which internal traits we master and which ones we express.

Know this: Successful people can identify a method that allows them to be successful and repeat it.

They are not hardworking some days, they are hardworking most days.

They are not delivering good customer service some days, they deliver it most days

They have good habits not some of the time, but most of the time.

Our goal must surely be to have a strong knowledge of our own internal ingredients. We must take meaningful action to build the traits we need and master the art of expressing the best and most appropriate ones in the pursuit of our goals.

We can break down your internal state into 9 CORE categories. Each core has its own sphere of influence over your life, and each core can unlock doors to creating results you might be missing out on.

The essence of this book is built around these 9 core internal systems. We are going to examine them 1 at a time. We are going to build a complete picture of who you are internally. It's going to be fun. Possibly to a glass of wine and some music? Possibly grab the yoga mat? Find your comfortable zone, and get the creative juices flowing, get the mind opened-up and get ready to spend some quality YOU time.

Engineering a new you will mean taking that evolutionary step towards the ideal you that shows up so often in your dreams. It's about time the two of you meet.

Before we launch off the diving board, I want to relay a story. While competing as a professional tennis player, it was imperative to always tweak, trying new things, experiment and search for the holy grail of improvement. I was trying very hard to be more balanced towards taking some risk on the bigger points. What this means is that I was a total scaredy pants. I literally became the deer in the headlights on my bigger opportunities. Saying that I had anxiety was an understatement.

My coach, to her eternal credit, knew that I was having a really hard time asserting myself, and so she made a deal with me, that I was only going to play assertively on ONE important point. Just one.

That's all.

Just one.

JUST ONE GODDAMMIT!!!

Like magic, that sentence opened something inside of me. A pathway to action. Of course, I could do it ONE time. Just because I was the most risk averse person on the face of the earth, and just because my hands were sweating so profusely new life forms were springing forth in the primordial soup collecting on my grip, and just because I couldn't form a cohesive thought if you hit me over the head with a wrench, I knew that I could do this ONE time.

For heaven sakes.

Come on man.

The key was making the goal small enough that there was: *just no way I could not do it.*

Why is that story important? Because there will be some of you that are absolutely terrified of taking the risk of messing with your self-perception. Scared to death of imagining what you could be. Not only does that make you confront your mistakes, but it also makes you confront your dreams head on, and then turn around and realize you haven't achieved them yet. If we can find some small way to move one of those needles by just a small amount, it can become the catalyst that slingshots you into the future. Because life is not just about knowing how you work, it's about finding a vision for how you MIGHT work.

We are not here to turn you into the next Michael Jackson, Warren Buffet, or have you moving to the Easter Island to live on a houseboat. What we are trying to do is look at some ways to practically help you.

Maybe you need to knock off 20 pounds. Let's lose 'em.

Maybe your idea is worthy of being built. Let's build it.

Maybe you have a relationship that is worth saving. Let's save it.

Maybe you have some beliefs that are holding you back. Let's ditch them.

Maybe you already do have an amazing life but are just too stressed to enjoy it. Let's ditch the stress.

Maybe you haven't dreamed of anything different for a while now. Let's dream just a little bit again!

Core 1: Your Overall State

Your overall state can be described as how you start your day off. Do you wake up with a lot of energy? Do you have a plan for the day? Do you get angry easily? Are you going to let traffic get you flustered? Do you anticipate problems? Do you have some solutions for them? Are you happy and excited to be alive?

We all have a basic set of emotions that are present all the time. We all have our distilled, key personality, whether that be fun-loving, serious, antsy, chatterbox, etc. This section aims to go through the "basic you" with a lens toward what your strengths are and what are some of the things that are holding you back.

To paint a picture of how these traits are combined in the most effective way, let's keep building on our example of Steve Jobs. He not only had the creativity to design and put together new products, he also could attract the right people from investors, to engineers to designers to marketers etc.

This shows he has excellent skills across a range of categories. Contrast this with someone who has incredible work ethic but lacks the creativity or the leadership and ends up merely being an employee for years.

Grab a comfy spot and get ready to think about how you perform in the following categories. Are you:

1. **Teachable**: This is a double-edged sword. My alpha personality, decision maker types, love to be in charge. They love to make the calls, so they are not always easy to teach. In reality, there are lessons you need to learn, and the teacher is not always your coach: it's your

results, your failures, your mentors, it's watching those around you. The question is-- do you learn? What lessons are taking you longer to learn than they should?

2. **Negative:** We can all fall victim to a negative mindset- particularly after a couple of setbacks. It is important to trust your process and make the effort to weed out negative thoughts. It's also important to understand how negativity can affect others and their productivity or group morale. What makes you negative? How quickly do you become negative?

3. **Motivated:** You need to have your WHY. If it's a strong one, you can stomach just about any process. We will need a good skill set and self-knowledge to understand what our internal, external, positive and negative motivators are- and how to keep the fire in the belly. Nothing can steal your motivation more than failure, and distractions. Be ready to confront those two things head on. What lights your candle? What gets you stoked? What gets you out of bed early ready to roll?

4. **Embrace Change:** Things Change. Things need to be changed. How comfortable are you with these concepts? Coaches quit. Relationships end. Companies go under. People get promoted ahead of you? Can you roll with it?

5. **Your Energy Management:** We talk here about the four quadrants; and where you fit in.

   1. High energy positive

   2. High energy negative

3. Low energy positive

4. Low energy negative.

High energy is probably key, and positive high energy beats out negative high energy, but a little negative can kick you into action faster than someone yelling "shark" when you are in the ocean. Which one are you? What's stopping you from taking more actions each day?

6. **Adaptable:** Life can throw you some major curveballs. You only have to be broke and about to lose the house once to see how resourceful you really are. You have to adapt. There are too many stories of the person who's company went under, or who's industry got usurped. Think of the folks who worked for Blackberry, or Nokia, or Blockbuster? Think of 2002 and 2008 stock market crash. You are going to get your rear end handed to you on a silver platter from time to time. You have to be ready to adjust and adapt to navigate your way back to the top. How adaptable are you?

7. **Patient:** When we speak of work/reward balance- life and business can be extremely unforgiving and can push this balance completely out of whack. You might have to works for months, sometimes years before you get the reward. You need a lot of confidence, and determination to keep doing this work at that level. Do you have realistic expectations? Can you be patient while building your future properly step by step?

8. **Diligent:** When the coach leaves you with 200 push-ups, 10 minutes jogging, and 10 other exercises- and then goes on to take an important phone call- do you

and the rest of the team do the work? OR do you slack off and discuss the week's latest soap opera? Does lack of confidence rob you of your ability to work without the reward for as long as it takes? Are you as diligent as an ant, as the saying goes?

9. **Attitude:** I have seen some people who are so good mentally, and work so hard and diligently, yet deep down they have a bad attitude. They have bad belief systems and they don't really believe things are going to end up well. Your underlying Attitude is everything, and it's something we need to work on all the time and keep it in healthy shape. What's your attitude like?

10. **Realistic:** Being realistic is important in terms of building lasting success. This does not mean have simple tiny goals. But it does mean that if you plan is to go to Vegas, and bet the house on red 33, then you are not being realistic about the chances of the risk working in your favor. I see people not realistic about the amount of training it takes to master a new skill. To carve out a new skill set takes a lot more than two sessions of 2 hours per week. 4 hours a week is a hobby, not something you are going to make opportunities out of. Does being realistic make you work your butt off, knowing that's what you need to do?

11. **Intensity:** Every successful person I have ever met has it. One of the emotions on this list they have in excess. Excess grit compared to peers. Excess determination. Excess ability to bounce back from failure. The intensity of these emotions is often what they use to become brilliant.

12. **Own the Love:** Do you love your sport or business because YOU love it? Do you do it because your parents force you, because you have nothing better to do. Are you passionate? We ask this question, because sheer love of what you do is going to come in very handy in some of the less rewarding parts of your career. There will be times when you and your art form are not jibing, if you know what I mean, but if deep down you feel grateful that this is your chosen profession, even on your worst days, that love is going to work wonders.

13. **Self-confidence:** Believe that it's possible, and that you are capable of doing it. Mastery of elements of this list is key to building internal belief structures that enable and empower breakthrough decision making and action taking. Develop good habits, good discipline, work ethic, and feed on a sense of accomplishment, and you will no doubt build the type of self-confidence that underpins results.

CORE NUMBER 2: ACTION INTERNALS.

Action.

Nothing great can get done without it.

You are what you do. Not what you say you do.

Do you jump out of bed and just take a massive amount of action?

I have seen some people over the years who could outwork a mule. I have also seen some people who could sleep through an FBI raid on their house, helicopters and all. What core internal systems are directing the how and when of your actions?

Have you nurtured and built up the right internals that allow you to take that critical step in the process of building a dream life: getting out there and actually doing it? Psychology texts are filled with reasons why humans take action, from needs and wants to impulses or fears, chemistry even. Successful people have almost all taken full control over their actions.

TIP: Don't forget: as you go through these, jot down what you would score yourself on a scale of 1 to 10

1. **Discipline:** Discipline maintains that you are going to do what you said you would, despite weather, distractions, girlfriends/boyfriends, losses, failure and anything else. We attach heavy value on this internal ingredient, because it keeps you moving forward better than any other value, except for maybe passion and love for what you do. Where are you on this scale? If you start a 12-week program-- are you absolutely going

to finish it? Do you prioritize your own goals above someone else?

2. **Work ethic:** One of your more important tools in life, period. The amount of work you are **capable of doing** and the amount of work you are **willing to do**, all will play a pivotal role in your future success. In no way does work ethic alone get the job done, there are still choices on how to direct that work. But when you break it down to brass taxes, are you someone who is comfortable with working hard?

3. **Competitiveness:** You have to know how to make things into a competition. You have to make your goals a challenge, give them a definitive timeline, fire up your competitive instincts, get resilient, make it happen. You have to know how to battle. I see so many talented people, who are just not that competitive- they think telling their bud at the gym of their invention is what's going to launch them into the stratosphere. When that doesn't work, they simply go back to their day jobs and let their dream sit in the corner. Are you willing to compete, face others on the same path? Others with more resources than you? Others with teams while you are a lone warrior? Does the idea of competing and coming out on top excite you? Are you a natural competitor?

4. **Fight:** One of the core components of your competitiveness is your ability to fight. This is something that is going to take you a long way in life. And if it's targeted towards the good of the world- then it's even better! If you roll over and fade into inactivity when challenged, then it's too easy to get you

to stop trying and go home. Are you a fighter? Can you dig down deep and find resources you never thought you had?

5. **Confidence**: Another huge topic, worthy of its own book. What we need to know is that confidence is a multifaceted beast. You need to be confident in yourself, you need to be confident in your method, you need to be confident in your team, and you also need to be wary of being delusional. These different confidences form a net of sorts. If you have very little self-confidence left after a string of losses, your confidence in your process can hold you up. You keep working because your discipline does not break down, and you end up rebuilding that lost performance confidence. Do you believe in yourself? Do you believe that a good method with real diligence can make a difference? Deep down, are you worthy of success?

6. **Creativity**: This is an important category- and it speaks to how you are thinking. Most creative people tend to understand that they need some kind of maze to design their way out of. Give them too much laundry and they will invent a washing machine. Someone who is not creative might get sulky, annoyed and into a limited resourcefulness state when confronted with a challenge. Even if you just look farther up this list, you have a vast array of emotional resources at your disposal, and it's up to you to be creative about how you use them. In fact, a huge part of what this journey we are on is about, is being **emotionally creative**. We could decide to have a war for example, or we could instead decide to find a common ground and build relationships with our neighbors-- the smartest people

emotionally are able to use their emotions incredibly constructively. Are you a creative problem solver? Are you ready to do this? Are you prepared for some unforeseen events that might be properly tough to overcome?

7. **Decisiveness:** Once you have made some considerations- can you be decisive? Funny enough I learned an important lesson here by accident. I started cramping deep into the third set tie-break, and decided I had no choice but to chip charge and come in. I would have agonized over that decision without the cramps- and would have played that tactic with a lot of doubt and hesitation (see earlier when I talk about my almost medical grade risk aversion). The cramps made it easy. I was decisive. I learned that you need to make your choice quickly, that way you can have all your reserves available for the actual execution. Step one is making a choice on direction, then step two is going out and executing. It's incredibly tough to execute if you are in two minds as to what it is you are trying to execute. Doubt, hesitation and baggage can slow down your reaction time, and inhibit your ability to access your skill. Are you decisive? Can you make some decisions and stick with them until the next check-point?

8. **Trust yourself:** After it has all been said and done, you have to trust yourself. Trust is something built over time through a large sample set. If you have been disciplined and hardworking, if you have consistently built yourself up adding layer upon layer of skill, then you will start to feel a deep-seated sense of self trust. If you have a history of making decisions that are

successful, then you will trust your decisions. Are you mired in doubt? Do you instantly see yourself quitting in week two, only to reinforce that you can't finish what you started? Do you trust that you will stay the course?

9. **Positive Output:** This is another area that's super important- and No, it does not mean you have to be smiling all the time. It means that you will be ready to fight, compete, hustle, show up on time, and work the goal hard. It means your output is building rather than destroying. That is worth its weight in gold. Are you ready to put some major positive, building, nurturing time into your goal?

10. **Concentration:** A skill which can be improved greatly with practice, the masters of concentration can get themselves into a deep state of absolute focus, from where they do their best work. Think of a surgeon here, think of an air traffic controller. We all know days that we are very distracted, versus days where we are not that distracted. Can you settle down into a rock-solid state of concentration?

11. **Tenacious:** Many a Business Deal has been pulled together on the fifteenth call, not on the first. Many a great accomplishment has happened because of the ability of the person to keep the idea alive in their mind, let go of embarrassment and call again. I have played some incredibly tough tenacious personalities in my life, and they all seem to have that one special quality: STAYING POWER. They hang around and hang around and eventually they find an opportunity. It's just a matter of time before they have a brilliant

day in the zone. It's just a matter of time before their opponent has a moment of lapse and makes a critical error. Very hopeful little fellas, my tenacious types. They really do believe they are on the brink of a breakthrough, and they just need to keep plugging away until they get it. Are you tenacious?

12. **Catalyst:** Thoughts and events that can spur you into action. Suddenly you see a pretty girl and you want to ask her out, so you decide to drop 10 pounds. A positive review, a promotion, a headhunter calls seeking your services. A new goal pops into your head. These are examples of catalysts, situations or a series of events that cause a chemical reaction inside of you, triggering alternate outcomes. The greats know how to trigger themselves, they know what their catalysts are. They keep the positive ones close, and the negative ones at bay. That powerful dream driving their motivation is close at hand, only a few thoughts away, and only a few seconds away from delivering a power surge in belief, in motivation and in action. How in touch are you with your catalysts?

Core 3: Your Ego/Self Satisfaction Internals.

The saying goes; "Don't let your EGO write a check that your body can't cash!"

Oh Yes! The good old EGO. A wonderful friend at times and your worst enemy at others. At its most basic, here we are dealing with what you think about yourself. What you believe you are entitled to. What you think you deserve. What type of a person you think you are? Your self-image. Your self-interest. The foundation of your morality. The drive and willingness to do just about anything to maintain a favorable view of yourself. The Ego can be a handy tool when you have built up a self-image that you strive to protect and it allows you to take supportive action towards your dream. It can be a nightmare when it does not allow you to make the right adjustments and thwarts your ability to learn and progress. Work through the following components, again scoring a 1-10 or making some notes as to where you feel strong or weak.

1. **Tolerate criticism:** If you really want to excel, you will need to face the negative stuff, and be able to hear the truth even though it hurts. Think about some of the paparazzi and how ruthless they can be with a bad performance from one of the stars. You need a thick skin, and you need to develop an appetite to want to know where you are weak.

   In fact, flip the script and purposefully seek out some harsh critics in the real world. One of the best examples of using criticism to the advantage of a business is the focus group. Designed to ask a million questions of a product or service, the whole idea is; In depth and detailed analysis and criticism of the product so you can make it better. You want to know the defects and shortcomings, and if you really do have a plan to work on them, this won't be threatening at all. If you are sitting still and have decided that this is who you are, then criticism will hurt a lot more. Can you take healthy criticism?

2. **Feel sorry for self:** Oh Yes! It can happen to the best of us, we get pouty and feel sorry for ourselves. The sooner you snap out of it, or better yet, stop doing it entirely, the better off you are. What we really need to watch out for here is justifying failure because of all the things happening 'TO YOU'. The traffic, your alarm broke, your lack of resources, and on and on the list goes. Can you avoid a "woe is me" attitude?

3. **Take position as a victim:** Although similar to feeling sorry for yourself, being a victim really is more about deferring responsibility. "He got lucky" "Life is always against me" The position that it is happening to you makes it easier to avoid responsibility, but unfortunately is a misguided perception of cause and effect.

4. **Spend energy on things you can't control:** Resources are often scarce. The resource of time is definitely scarce, and therefore we need to choose how to use it wisely. Some things you can't control. Some things you can. You have to decide whether moaning about whatever it is, is productive, or whether you should accept it and focus on your something you can influence instead. Can you discern quickly things

worthy of your time, and things that no amount of action will influence, therefore you should let them go?

5. **Try to please everyone:** you will have a lot of people vying for your attention, and you will need to know what your priorities are. This will inevitably mean that you will have to learn to say NO! Learn how to do this, early on!

6. **Entitled:** Generally, this means you feel like you should get stuff just because you are you. The balance between having earned something, or even if the need is rational or not come into play here. I have seen some people storming around freaking out that their manicurist didn't have a certain type of glitter polish. This was enough to call management and try to have the person fired. Generally, being entitled stems from an exaggerated sense of self, it normally saps motivation and work ethic, and can break down your ability to achieve as you start to expect results without doing the work. It can also spell disaster for future planning, as believing you are entitled to a certain lifestyle may make it hard to adjust up and down as your resources demand.

7. **Instant gratification:** I want it. I want it now. Impulsiveness. This can cause you a myriad of problems. From overtraining, (because 9 hours per day must be better than six and will get me there faster) to poor, impulsive decision making based entirely on what will make you feel gratified right now. Compulsion stems from this state. Countless journeys have been stopped because the person wanted results sooner than they actually come. Countless people have

literally been on the brink of success, only to stop or turn around at the last minute because they wanted results sooner. The truth is it can be incredibly difficult to predict when results will come, or when breakthroughs will happen. We should try to use common sense and historical precedents as leading indicators. These 12 week get-rich-quick schemes take advantage of the type of mentality that believes they can outfox the system and achieve things in one 10th of the time it takes other people. In reality, you most likely will have to work hard and stay the course for a longer period of time than you originally thought, to actually get there. Of course, the ideal scenario is that you simply love what you are doing, and success is simply an extension of a lifestyle you love. How many people have decided to do a job they don't like because they wanted the rewards of it, and were willing to sacrifice their lifestyle, only to wake up 20 years later, and realize they are still broke, and wasted 20 years on something they don't even like?

8. **Seek attention:** This is an interesting one. It is important to know if getting attention is one of your drivers. You have no real passion for the item, your reward is attention. Stop getting the attention and watch how quickly the love of the sport or idea drops. Recognition is good, but there have to be a number of other drivers present other than getting acknowledgement from others. How important is this to you? Take a second to think it through and grade yourself 1-10.

9. **Overreact:** We have all overreacted at one point in another in our lives. A flood of emotion leading to a

reaction out of proportion with the size of the situation. Repetitive over reacting could mean a recalibration of your emotional system is required. Perhaps you are carrying some baggage from a previous situation that needs to be attended to.

Let's use an example of someone who gets too aggressive, Bob. Bob gets cut off in traffic. It upsets him. A huge surge of adrenaline is followed by telling the other driver exactly which station in life he can get off at.

Problem is, in the adrenaline-fueled emotional drama, Bob forgets to pick up the newly printed exhibits for his client meeting at 9 am. The potential client feels that Bob is unprepared and naturally, the deal walks out the door with them. Yes, Bob overreacted and yes, it was expensive.

10. **Need Reward:** This is an interesting one. Do you need the reward to have the discipline? We look at so many former athletes and once the competition is gone, so are they. They just have to have that next week's prize of playing the tournament to keep them motivated, keep them taking action. There has to be something on the line. Ask yourself if you can do the hard yards just because they are there to be done, or if you need a trophy or some other type of reward. Think of it neither as a good thing nor a bad thing, but more a matter of practicality. If you do need a reward, plan one in your system, or seek out environments that offer them. Just don't find yourself languishing with no motivation because you are in an environment that

offers no reward, yet the reward is the missing driver of performance that you need.

11. **Perfectionist:** A valuable tool for sure but a double-edged sword. Perfectionists will go to great lengths to make sure something is just right, and that's a huge bonus. Where it can be a problem is that things so seldomly go perfectly. Perfectionists can be quite easily rattled and frustrated, and this can derail them. Is trying to be perfect driving you crazy?

12. **Ethics:** Being a good person is important to me. It should be important to you. There are some mega successes that are ethically a zero. Think Pablo Escobar here. Not only is becoming a billionaire through his method requiring of a moral makeup that is completely out of whack, you also have all the brilliant side-effects like running from the cops, building safe-houses, and evading the FBI to deal with. Think about how your ethics feed back into your ego and self-esteem.

13. **Humility/Appreciative:** You need to be able to stop and smell the roses. You have to work on that feeling of deep gratefulness that you are inside a human body right now, able to do this thing you love and able to compete and have your chance to manifest a dream to reality. So very few people have this chance, and its absolute bliss to be a human for 80 years until 'poof', its gone. Knowing and understanding this is a key part of being able to stay the course. If you never forget how lucky you are, even your worst days are endowed with a silver lining.

I believe emphatically, biblically even, that no growth is meaningful until you know what you are comparing it with. It becomes invaluable when that comparison keeps you humble.

14. **Dwell on mistakes:** You are going to blow it! There will be times where it's completely your fault, you absolutely made the wrong call, and you blew it. Months of hard work, whole team excited and relying on you, and you wreck it! Its savage. Your guts are shredded. Do you lock yourself in a room for months, and cry through 1000 boxes of Kleenex, or do you own it, start the necessary fall-out clean up, and get back to forward progress as soon as possible?

18. **Associations:** What do you associate with cool? What do you associate with success? False associations, as any of the cigarette smoking whiskey swilling dudes from the fifties will tell you, can lead to chasing the wrong goals, and taking actions that serve no purpose other than to hurt you and your body, rather than facilitate a legacy of awesomeness. Check your associations. Regularly.

Core Number 4: Thick Skin Internals.

This is one of my favorite core segments. This is the group of internal attributes that will steer you around, through, over or simply obliterate the obstacles. These are the ones that allow you to suck it up, dust off and come back for more. Rocky Balboa style. The human being is capable of incredible feats of hanging in there, of staying until the job is done, and these internals are the ones that make reaching the finish line possible. Millions of people are left with 'what if's?' and 'maybe's' because they fell short in the thick skin department. Take a look at the accomplishments of Martin Strel: Marathon River swimmer. This fella swam the Amazon. The whole thing. Got hit by lightning, chomped on by piranhas. He kept going. Would you go back in the water after piranhas took a little snack bite out of your upper back?

We spoke earlier about your level of commitment, your level of GO button. This whole set is based on 'gut-check' time.

Read through this set of internals, and grade yourself 1-10.

1. **Sacrifices:** In order to excel at one thing, you have to take time away from something else. Whether that be Nintendo, your breakdancing class, or your weekly trip to the lake. Generally something needs to give, in order for you to spend more time on the dream. There are many people who kinda-sorta want it, but they don't want it more than their Facebook time, their mall time, their social Saturday time. There is a big question that only you can answer: How bad do you want it?

2. **Persistence:** The dictionary describes persistence as: "obstinate continuance in a course of action, despite difficulty or opposition." Are you the type of person who is going to keep coming back? Keep re-inventing? Developing new tools. Do you have a lot of persistence when it comes to implementing them? Trying them? Persistence requires an acute understanding of the need to evolve, and an ownership of the idea that you have to keep refining, adapting and getting better.

3. **Resiliency:** Best you stock up double on this one. Depending on your field, you are going to take some beat downs. Some of them are going to sting. Like, emotional equivalent of a box jelly fish, sting. If you consist of flabby, fragile mental mush, those beat downs are going to make you want to quit. You are going to face "The WALL" many times, a blockage so severe it seems there is no reasonable way around it. In fact, the number one reason people quit is because the beatdowns destabilize them too much: they hit at your confidence, they hit at your motivation, they hit at your will. You need to train your WILL to where it is like a cockroach in a nuclear disaster. The radiation can knock out just about every other living thing, but the cockroach somehow finds a way to stay alive. I have seen people lose everything, the cars, the millions, the fame. They suffer public (and private humiliation) and yet, you cannot kill their WILL.

4. **Pain Tolerance:** You're going to want to stock up on both **Emotional** pain tolerance as well as **Physical** pain tolerance. You are going to cry, lose control, get angry, experience deep frustration. You are going to go

to places emotionally that other people will not. You are going to go to physical places that other people will not. You are going to open doors to rooms in your mind where your deepest fears and inadequacies are lurking. You might need to slay some dragons, my friend. It's going to be legendary! You are going to feel spectacular when you are done.

5. **Grit:** Sandpaper. Velcro. Clingy static electricity. Stick to the task like feathers to super glue. It's never a linear path to anything. You are going to get derailed, you are going to get shut down, you are going to get sledgehammered to the ground. Grit is that pesky personality trait that makes you shrug it off and keep going. Clench the teeth, grin and bear it baby!

6. **Self-reliant:** When you are in the heat of battle, no-one can decide what to do next but you. Again, you can train and train and train, but the crucial decisions that change outcomes are up to you. Have you built yourself into someone who can make these decisions and rely on yourself here?

7. **Embrace Failure**: A lot of times it's the things we are not good at that stick out-- I have seen some people who really can bounce back fast. They embrace failure, are able to learn from it, and make their next attempt a good one. The idea is that the real wealth is in the opportunity. Creating a lot of them for yourself is the real prize. If you only create one opportunity for yourself ever, the amount of pressure to "seize this ONE moment ever in your life" will be almost unbearable. Realistically, if your future is dependent on one deal coming through, or this one test, you

probably have a lot of missing ingredients. A good method and process will generate many opportunities for you. If you miss one or two, no need to panic, you will make another one for yourself. Those who have an iron clad PROCESS, work ethic dialed in, and clear goals, are almost always just around the corner from another opportunity. Can you move on, or are you still talking about the time you nearly scored a touchdown in 6th grade?

While we all want the nice comfortable life, and we are taught to fear discomfort, the reality is that growth often comes from very emotionally tough places. Those big break ups, those huge losses, those missed opportunities can strengthen your resolve, and force you to grow in ways you never could without them. So often failure is a mirror that show you where you went wrong. All too often, we try and convince ourselves that what we are seeing in the mirror is not correct, and that the mirror is actually wrong. If you can switch off the ego, and take a proper look, failure is one of your best and most honest teachers. Annoying, and someone you often disagree with, failure is in fact a little mini Yoda that you will want to listen to.

8. **Emotional Range:** We all have our own emotional comfort zone. We have developed tolerances for certain feelings, we function just fine within them. Go outside of that range and we start to feel uncomfortable. Of course, that uncomfortable feeling makes you go right back into your nice warm, cuddly little comfort zone. In order to really grow a thick skin, we are going to need to operate in a far greater range than we are accustomed to. You will experience some

emotion on your way to excellence. Expect some crankiness, anger, frustration, sadness, bewilderment, serious pushing and a whole host of feelings that you don't normally subject yourself to, to become a part of your new daily experience.

CORE NUMBER 5: WISDOM INTERNALS.

Experience is the mother of wisdom. Failure is the mother of experience. If you want to get wise early, then you want to fail a lot, early on. Learn from those failures. Learn enough and you will start to become wise. When you get to the point where you are making internal and external choices based on wisdom, then you can start to cut out a lot of the messy, mistake-learn-try again-fail again cycle. Good judgement is something we should all strive for. Wisdom is the antidote to being an idiot! This core group speaks to your wisdom, and your relationship with the items in this subset will go a long way towards delivering you to your personal promised land.

1. **Taking Risk:** Another topic that we need a whole book to go through. In order to truly excel, you have to place your bets. Like any stock market winner, you will never have that huge success story unless you make the investment in Facebook, or Microsoft, or Bitcoin, or whichever stock goes quadruple platinum. You will need to be able to make that move and put your money in the middle. The how, why, and which risks should be taken, that is the art form. People, classes, ideas. Place your bets and make your choices as to which endeavors are best suited to invest your time into.

2. **Moderating risk:** Just as being willing to take some risk is important, being able to moderate that risk is absolutely critical. Maybe you sit down to write a book and decide to put 40 hours a week into it. You decide to rather be a bit tired instead of quitting your day job,

better to be a little cranky and sleep deprived than homeless. Naturally, if you are able to moderate risk well, you will develop a healthy risk balance, and this can be a hugely important weapon.

3. **Problem solving:** You don't know what you don't know. Trial and error takes time, and many tries. While we are grunting and swearing and having a fat tantrum, groaning our way to success, the wise person makes the right decision for the situation. You are thinking: 'Lucky bastard!" You need to really understand your area of expertise to be able to be a great problem solver, and studying, learning, acquiring that high level is a must. The 10,000 hours: DO THEM. You want to be the expert!

4. **Decision making:** This is a huge and complex topic, and certainly deserves its own long methodological approach to understanding. The questions you want to ask are: "Am I am good decision maker? Am I impulsive? Do I over analyze? Are my decisions to avoid discomfort? Are they to minimize friction? Do I have a process for how I make decisions? Am I flexible enough to change those decisions? What is the evidence I need to make those changes?

5. **Emotional Intelligence:** No matter which way you slice it, you are going to make decisions based on your emotions all the time. With practice, you are supposed to be improving. The problem is, a lot of people keep making the same emotional errors! We want to evolve into a highly sophisticated emotional being. And as the athletes will tell you, practice does not make perfect, it

makes permanent. Only perfect practice makes perfect. So, it's time to start practicing those emotions!!

6. **Multi-tasking: A Game within a game:** This is an often-understated skill set but is worth its weight in gold. We all have a girlfriend or mother in law who is absolutely brilliant at it. Phone in one hand, kid in the other, chopping vegetables in some mysterious way that no one has ever figured out, and all the while telepathically sensing mathematical questions and to yelling homework answers to a child sitting in another room. Working on a number of things simultaneously is going to increase your productivity. Learn how to do it, learn how to spot opportunities, albeit small ones, to chip away at other tasks and get them done.

7. **Reason vs Emotion:** Do you make your decisions based on reason or emotion? More importantly- when you are extremely emotional, how good is your decision making? We spoke earlier about your emotional range, and how some people don't get that stressed. But lack of panic can also lead to lack of action.

8. **Pick your battles: I have two great examples here.** Midway through his career, Federer ran into this fella named Nadal. He decided to try and play Nadal at his own game, trying to outlast him. Trying to out-grind him. This was a mistake, and it took him many losses to finally admit that he picked a fight with the wrong guy, or more importantly, he picked the wrong type of fight with that guy. Just recently, he decided to play his naturally aggressive style, but build his backhand into a far more capable shot against Nadal. (Please take a

note here: this is taking one of the best backhands the world has ever seen, and making it better, something most of us would not consider.) This is a great example of how the best think.

CORE NUMBER 6: PEOPLE INTERNALS.

No one is self-made. That concept that is a logical fallacy. Think of your teachers at school, parents, friends, mentors and all the people you interact with along the way. Finally, there will be the client, person who is buying your product or service, listening to your music, reading your book (wink-wink) You need to have people skills, you need to know how to work with people, get the best out of people, motivate people. If you have genuine empathy for people, genuinely care for their best outcomes and have designed products that solve problems and add value, then you are going to do extremely well in this world. Here are some of the core people internals. Grade yourself 1-10.

1. **Leadership**: You need to be one, and you need friends and supporters who are good ones. It's imperative that you learn to lead your teammates into good practices and are able to build and maintain highly competitive practices, contributing to an excellent culture.

2. **Able to sense and react to other's emotions:** Emotionally smart people can sense when the other person is about to do something silly. They can sense when recklessness is on the table. They can sense when will and resolve are fading and can make excellent judgements about the other person's emotions. They

can sense when fear and anxiety are at their peak. They can see when someone is emotionally tired. They know when to push, when to be patient, when to dig the heels in, when to attack.

3. **Build great team around yourself:** No-one can do it alone, and you need good people around you. Make sure to build that team, and build the character traits, attributes, standards and methodology that the team adheres to.

4. **Whining and complaining;** This really is about management. You only have a certain amount of time. It's like a bank balance. If you spend your cash on junk, then you probably won't have much left over for investing. If you spend your time moaning and complaining, then you probably won't have that much left over for finding solutions. There is a need for emotional venting, but realistically, this happens occasionally, not all the time. The best in the world invest in positive self-talk, they talk about solutions, the self-coach. And, they secretly love the problems. They enjoy being the one who solved them, or the one who had the cool calm demeanor while everyone was having a meltdown the equivalent of Fukushima and Chernobyl having a lovechild.

5. **Are you a control freak:** Great for training, preparation, organizing flights and making things happen. Bad for letting other people do their jobs. Have to tame this trait with an acute knowledge of the things you can't control. Have to know that you are quite average, bordering on horrible at certain things, and that's why you PAY or ask others to help you get them done. Michael Jackson's agent still makes millions, but you won't see him take the microphone any time soon. If you can be a control freak who is in control of the things you can have an impact on- then you will do extremely well.

6. **Blame others:** Do heads roll in your team when you don't get the result you want? This can make it tough to build loyalty, if people feel like they might get the chop anyway. Most importantly, it can be tough to take the necessary corrective steps if you can't look in the mirror and admit it is YOU who needs to change.

7. **Honest:** You have to be honest with yourself. Are you willing to change? Are you willing to put in the hard work? Are you willing to face your fears? Are you willing to go the distance?

8. **Dependable:** No Doubt this is a valuable asset. People can trust you, and you can trust you. You show up. You bring your core emotional set with you. You can be relied upon.

CORE NUMBER 7: PERFORMER INTERNALS

Not all jobs have the performer aspect to them. But for those that do- (think public speaking, acting, tennis player, salesperson, trial lawyer, surgeon) you need to develop the skills to be able to perform well. As a former professional tennis player, I can certainly attest to how difficult it is to do something in a match versus doing it in practice. I can attest to how difficult it is to come up with a great idea in the heat of the moment. We have probably all had a situation where we meet someone, and only when we are back in the car after the meeting do we think "I totally should have said this" or "I should have asked this" Unfortunately the moment has passed. Great performers tend to think their best in the heat of the battle. I have a good friend who is a legendary salesperson in the medical devices arena, and I have been with him on a number of sales appointments as part of my research and preparation for this book. He has to field off so many questions and explain so many different details on each call that he really has to be on the top of his game. Break it down to brass taxes, and your performer skills are the summation of your training, and the part where you go out there and actually DO it. Working as a coach, I spend an enormous amount of time in this category, because there are so many things that can influence your performance. Nerves, stress, low confidence, slow reactions, indecisiveness. I was able to maintain a winning record of around 60% for my tennis career, all based on good performer internals. This was not always the case, I had a number of awful performance runs in junior tennis. I tended to get down on myself, I tended to be extremely over cautious, and I tended to lack direction. This led to becoming frustrated and emotional, losing my temper and of course losing a lot of matches. I learned over the years to find a deeper state of concentration, and to manage risk in a more businesslike way. I learned to expect the nerves and have a plan for how to deal with them, rather than be emotional and resentful that they were there. I learned the value of preparation. Starting well could often put the opponent on the back foot right away and keep them emotionally off balance for the remainder of the match. I learned that you CANNOT predict the future, and you do not know when your next opportunity will come. I decided to fight for every point, for the entire duration of my matches. I learned to deploy positive self-talk and support my own dreams. I used a lot of positive affirmations. Let's sift through the more important ones on the list of being a great performer

1. **Progress versus regress**: This is a huge one- What do your forward steps look like versus your backward steps? I have seen some remarkable achievements from people who just plod along, taking only a little bit of ground at a time, but not giving much if any back. If you add a couple of bricks per day, and never take any out, you will be amazed at what you can build in 10 years! Injury, Life events can all step in and make themselves annoyingly known. But the focus here is on things we can control. The great performers are always looking for progress. They have learned to hold on to

any inches gained. Take a trip to the Grand Canyon, and you will notice that you can remove a whole lot of rock with steady constant progress.

2. **Decisions under pressure:** How good of a decision maker are you under pressure? If you find yourself in an emergency situation, will you come up with logical decisions? Are you instinctively good at making decisions under stress or do you need to follow some kind of plan to arrive at your decisions? If yes, how do you formulate this plan?

3. **Ability under pressure:** Many a brilliant opportunity had been squandered by the person only being able to use a tiny fraction of their actual skill when it matters. Many a performer has frozen in the spotlight and is simply unable to access their best stuff when it matters. Nervous energy, tension, the fight or flight instinct and muddled decision making simply overwhelm the body and mind. It's like sugar in the gas tank, you splutter and gasp, but inevitably are unable to perform. We need to put a lot of work into this piece, because it's one of the more vital ones on this list

4. **Ability to show up:** this is not just speaking to your reliability. This is also speaking to YOU, at full power, full competitiveness showing up for battle. Intense, fortified, and ready to be a baller? Are you the one who shows up emotionally day in and day out, week in and week out?

5. **Repeat Mistakes:** This is one that takes some introspection. Think about the things you have bumped your head against the wall about multiple times. Do you always go into high risk mode when

things get close- you just want it to end- fast-no matter what the outcome? Knowing whether you won or lost is better than being in that highly stressed situation for another minute. Do you always become timid and hope the other person is going to miss? Do you always get angry in the same situation? Do you always quit given the same situation? It's difficult to identify emotional mistakes, but some of them are relatively easy to spot. Quitting is never a good choice. Sagging shoulders, poor body language.

6. **Emotional Response:** This means you can sense danger. You can sense complacency. You get upset at yourself if you feel yourself slacking. You immediately shore up risk if you feel yourself losing grit. You respond. If the person at the mall hits the deck, you are first on scene yelling "get me the defibrillator, get me 911". You respond. When one of your dreams comes under threat, so you sit and let the vultures pick at it, or do you respond?

7. **Can Commit full mind body spirit**: The ability to fully engage and get present, draw on your intellectual, physical and inspirational resources. "I kinda-sorta want to change my life" is a wishy-washy, one toe in the water approach to getting things done. When you have decided that you are in, ALL IN, and are willing to go the distance, come hell or high water, you are going create change.

8. **Impulse Control:** We all have certain impulses under pressure. At its most basic form, we will have two roads. The impulse to be passive or to play safe or the impulse to try and be aggressive and make the move

first. Both of these ideas have merit, but they also have problems. Understanding if you are naturally risk seeking or risk avoiding in critical moments is key to understanding your tactics and abilities under pressure.

9. **Self-Preservation/Survival instinct**. The human body is designed to survive. We are equipped with a monumentally powerful will to endure and live, and we don't need to look too far into a google search to find a story of someone who went to enormous lengths to survive. When you are performing, and you are threatened, it helps tremendously if your self-preservation and will to live kicks in. And this means that you need to care about stuff. If you care about outcomes, you will fight for them. If you are an iceberg and they don't affect you, it's unlikely that you will be able to reach in and tap into this most powerful of human emotions. This is the one internal trait can bring you about as close to supernatural ability as any on this list.

CORE NUMBER 8:
BUSINESSMAN/PROFESSIONALISM INTERNALS.

Being a pro. Professional. You show up on time. You meet your deadlines. People know and can trust you will do what you say you are going to do. You can separate the homelife from work and don't air your dirty laundry all over the show. You don't throw the stapler at your co-workers. You are the real deal. You attend to the details, and you can get the job done. Your professionalism stems from decisions made on how you want to go about your business. If you have made the decision to be at the top of your game in terms of how you dress, how you speak to and deal with your team and co-workers. If you are someone who takes the time to write the thank you card-remember the birthday. Show up early. Set up the equipment before your clients arrive. Well groomed, smelling good. Research done. Presentation beautiful. Known for not cancelling appointments at the last minute. Take care of the details, even the ones you don't like doing. You stay current- go to the conferences, do the continuing education. You are highly competent, you have built and execute the high level of skills to get the job done. You respect protocols and systems. You respect yourself and your teammates. You are a PRO my friend. Let's go through my top list of ones that I thought made the biggest difference

1. **Productivity:** Time is a valuable asset. Organizing how you will spend it is a little bit like squeezing a lemon. Some people really know how to get all the

juice out of it. You want to be that person. This takes planning, and it takes a keen eye for sidestepping distractions. Planning, focus, attention to detail and an overall attitude of wanting to get a lot done.

2. **Contemplation/Analysis:** In order to be an excellent tactician, you need to be smart. You need to make good choices. Someone who takes the time to contemplate, analyze, bring to the table new ideas, is going to do well. Some folks are like a bull in a China shop, they are extremely action based. Make sure to have someone on the team that is a thinker. Take pride in developing your ability to reason.

3. **Responsible:** Set goals. Make good choices. A huge part of being a pro and building your reputation is to be the responsible one. Take notes, write it on your hand, just be the person who delivers.

4. **Habit forming:** The golden word in excellence is PROCESS. In fact-by now you should understand the principle that your results are merely a reflection of your method. Your method of performing your skill set, your method of decision making, your method of eating, sleeping, thinking, technical improvement, body language, self-communication. If you are continually growing your method, adjusting and refining it- you end up with an incredible process. Trust me, if you develop an incredible method- people will notice and you become the go-to person to get things done.

5. **Set goals:** This is one we are going to dedicate a whole chapter to. For now, you need to think of your goals as the blueprint- Without them you will be surviving on chance a lot more than you will good planning. This

process is critical to bring into the conscious mind all the little steps that might be necessary to build something big.

6. **Organization skills:** Sadly, there are too many people who cannot organize their day well. I get it. Kids, doctors' appointments, car checkups, basketball practice, your squash game, date night, and on and on the list goes. On top of this, you still need to be the outperformer. There is only one way you can make this happen. You need to learn to organize. You need to have a master task list and tick little boxes. You need to stay one step ahead of the game. From this day forward- the word Logistics has taken on new importance.

7. **Consistency:** It's easy to set high standards for a week, or a month. The best can deliver their exacting, performance driven high standards over a long period of time. Your job is to build the Mercedes Benz of professionalism. You deliver. Consistently. Reliably. Time and time again. People can set their clocks by you.

8. **Build up others.** Pros are very good at getting the best out of the people around them. They have balanced the ego to where they can give credit to others when due. They can create opportunities for others. They support and cheer on their team.

CORE 9: POSITIVE COPING

One of the decisive elements in deciding if you will be able do something is your ability to cope with it. For most of us, we have a difficult time in being able to cope with our normal lives, so the idea of throwing something extra into the mix means that our already-stretched-to-the-limits system is not going to hold up.

Coping mechanisms equate to our internal ability to endure. Think of positive coping skills as the internal tools that give us our capacity to ride things out for the long haul.

Persistence. Grit. Keep going. Take the blows. Endure. At their core, they are all built around the same root: the ability to cope.

Can you cope with the early morning workouts?

Can you cope with the insane hours of medical school?

Can you cope with the hunger when trying to diet?

Can you cope with trying to break out of a poor self-perception?

No matter what it is you are trying to achieve, you will need to learn how to cope with the changes and the duties of your new endeavor. Let's explore how coping mechanisms work, and which ones help or hinder performance.

Evolution has equipped us with some extremely useful coping mechanisms, and it's important for us to be able to use them as and when needed to accomplish the things we set out to. Well trained, coping mechanisms become powerful tools. Poorly trained, coping mechanisms become a road to regression.

If you do not develop the correct coping mechanisms, you will undoubtedly fail. It is imperative that you do not look at this failure as a definitive end point, but rather an opportunity to build better coping strategies, and experiment with different ways of enduring the problem.

One way to frame this argument is to know that you have already learned how to cope. Many of us have learned to cope with a life of not achieving your dreams, of mediocrity, no new surprises. That's actually much more difficult to endure than a fun exciting adventure filled life, because the adventure itself provides much of the motivation.

Put differently, there is the potential you and the real you. For most of us, we have not reached our full potential, and there are many productive things we need to do in order to start opening up those doors to quantum level, exponential growth. Settling or coping with a you that's second rate is not the right way to use coping as a tool. Adjusting to new dreams, new ideas and new actions, and then learning to cope with those→ now that's the ticket! Our goal through this section is to turn the literature on its head and use all these known coping mechanisms in an applied way as a weapon to further our own development.

The self-image link to coping.

We need to have a small discussion regarding self-image. Your self-image tends to hold you prisoner to a number of behaviors. Marry that to other people holding you to their image of you, and you can see why breaking out and forging a new you can be a difficult. All too often we come across someone who has all the power and potential to achieve much more than they do. They have the opportunities, they have the skill set, but they simply do not see themselves as worthy, or as actually achieving the goal. Their self-esteem has handcuffed them to their current situation.

Self-esteem is an incredibly powerful mechanism. What you think of yourself will absolutely shape your outcomes, your decisions and ultimately your destiny.

In order for real growth to come, you will need to cultivate your self-image. Grow it and nurture it, feed it and look after it and become an obsessively good caretaker of it.

We all have a story that we have made up of who we are. That story most definitely can be changed, but it takes time and work and it is not normally a one stop journey to acceptance. Knowing this and realizing this is a key element in maintaining the dedication and discipline of robust self-image care.

Here are some of the most common coping mechanisms:

1) **Aim inhibition:** Lowering your sights and dreams to ones that seem more achievable.

The gap between wanting and not having causes tension. Rather than this tension being a positive motivating experience, this tension can be really stressful. Aim inhibition seeks to remove this uneasy feeling by reducing the goal and therefore minimizing the gap between outcomes you want and outcomes you already have. If you ever see someone who is way out of their comfort zone, and visibly struggling- look out for aim inhibition as their solution. It's very difficult to raise your sights if the mere idea of creating want is uncomfortable, and you instantly snuff it out.

2) Rationalization: Finding logical reasons why your behavior or lack thereof is justified.

When something happens that we feel is distasteful, we make up logical reasons why it happened. If we have stopped actively pursuing a goal, we logically rationalize why we have done so. If someone has been unkind to us, we find a way to rationalize this. We often rationalize our behavior as fitting into models, values and beliefs. When we do something that our moral superego disapproves of, then we begin the process of rationalization. This way we can do something truly awful and not feel to guilty about it. Our need for esteem also is a big reason why we will rationalize to complete strangers. The bully rationalizes what they have done by saying that the victim deserved it. In persuasion, offer people logical reasons why they can comply with your arguments. Explaining what happens creates consistency between actions and thoughts. For our intents and purposes, we need to rationalize our new behaviors, rationalize the discomfort we are feeling trying to keep our new habits in check- in other words, make sure you know your WHY!

3) Fantasy: Sometimes when we do not have or cannot achieve the things we want, we escape into a world of fantasy.

Think of the athlete who fails, who then says something like "I could have won if I really wanted to, but I was working on my slice backhand today." If you cannot afford the nice car, we fantasize about having it as a substitute to actually having it. Fantasy is a normal part of the human make-up, but of course the danger lies in enjoying the fantasy so much that we settle for it instead of the real thing. We want to avoid delusional obsessions, but draw energy and motivation from the "what if's?" When you are at the precipice of taking an action and you are being held back, possibly losing confidence and belief, or regressing to an old habit, a great trigger is to be able to imagine the future, imagine yourself pushing through, imagine some fun future outcomes if you stick with what you are doing. If you think about some of the people who for years worked without reward, they obviously had a good imagination as their way of keeping them going through the hard times.

4) Intellectualization: Avoiding emotion by focusing on logic and facts

At its core, the tactic here is to try and suppress emotion. By isolating or disconnecting the emotions surrounding an event, one can protect against anxiety. Powerful jargon and heightened or complex terminology are all symptoms of using intellectualization as the method of understanding or describing the problem. If you see someone in trying to go through a difficult situation in a cold unemotional way, they are most likely not ready to deal with the emotions and process them correctly.

5) Extreme Emotionality: Outbursts of extreme emotion.

When we become stressed, a number of negative emotions can start to build. Think jealousy, anger, fear and frustration. When we display these emotions, it generally affects those around us. Most cultures have a social contract that says we should not distress others, so these outbursts can create very negative opinions and results in your community. This, of course is the reason a lot of people bottle up their stress. If you put a high value on team and building the core group of people around you, it is hugely important to focus on releasing these feelings is a controlled, productive way.

6) Substitution: Replacing one activity for another.

The main idea here is to take something that leads to discomfort and replace it with something that does not lead to discomfort. Instead of making the tough phone call, we call a buddy and have a grand old conversation about the NFL instead. The common phrase here is putting off something we don't want to do. Procrastination and other forms of avoidance are all types of substitution. This coping mechanism can lead to vastly diminished outcomes. It's an application of the pleasure and pain principle, moving away from pain and towards pleasure, but the real problem here is that often your 'pain' is actually just perceptual, and once you start doing the thing you were avoiding, you find out it's much easier and more enjoyable than you thought. Then you start kicking yourself, thinking about all the other things that were just 'too difficult to do' that you have spent your whole life avoiding.

7) Conversion: Converting mental stress into physical actions-

One of the world's greatest coping mechanisms, the human being has the ability to convert mental stress into action. We have all heard the world's best all talk about how the heat of the moment "gets them going." What they are actually saying is that the stress of the moment makes them want to act. They immediately start to eliminate stress by taking the necessary steps to make things better. This is your golden zone, your mecca of coping, because you actually are spurred into action- the right action. Now, if you find yourself sitting in the corner of your house, having just eaten al of your finger nails off, and plucking your eyelashes out one by one... you might be using conversion the wrong way.

8) Regression: Return to pre-new habit state to avoid dealing with change.

The pleasure-pain principle at work again. There is familiarity in our old lifestyle and our old behaviors. The human body does not like stress. It reacts to it in many different ways, but the consistent theme is to return to a less stressed state. We do this through our various coping mechanisms. When we begin to feel stressed, it is very easy for our body to rationalize returning to the life we know, that we are comfortable with, that has worked and kept us safe from harm for so long. That silky voice of mediocrity has an alarming success rate of causing perfectly rational people to give up, give in and go back to the very thing they have spent so much energy and resolve trying to break free from. Think of the famous Stockholm syndrome- where you actually start developing positive feelings for your kidnappers- sticking up for them and justifying their behaviors. This is no different. Mediocrity is holding you captive, its kidnapped your potential and regression is a way of sticking up for your captor.

10) Rituals: A set of predetermined activities that you do before the stressful event.

Need to make a tough phone call, grab the notepad, write down your 5 key items you want to talk about. Go to washroom and brush teeth. Use mouthwash. Practice saying hello 30 times into mirror. If this sounds like you, then you have experience with the use of a ritual. Rituals are prescribed by many sports psychologists as a way to sift through the stress, avoid impulsive decisions, and train the habit mechanism. These predetermined activities give us just a little bit longer to think through the situation, to wait for the strong emotions to subside, and then make better decisions once the huge jolt of emotion in the situation has passed. Rituals keep feeding back signals that you are in control, and that you are the boss out there. They can have a very strong psychologically calming and stabilizing effect.

11) Compensation: Making up for weakness in one area by compensating with another.

The idea here is that when confronted with a weakness, you can say- "yes I am pretty bad here, but I am strong here", and so can avoid feeling bad about the weakness by immediately focusing on your strengths.

12) Introjection: The broad definition is to take something from the outside world and then make it our own.

The concept is to cope with needing to grow by finding people who have already solved a problem and learning from them. We live in a time where many things have already been achieved. This means that somebody, somewhere, has already achieved what you are trying to achieve. This also means that someone has figured out how to cope with what you are trying to cope with. Instead of trying to re-invent the wheel, have a look around and see how other people are coping with their successes and failures. Just repeating the mantra "someone else has successfully dealt with this" is normally enough to snap you out of feeling sorry for yourself and making the excuse that this is just too tough, and get you thinking there must be a solution. When you feel stressed, think of someone who handles the situation like a BOSS. Think like them, be like them and handle your challenge like James Bond would.

13) Diminishing. The idea here is to make something daunting in your mind seem much less so by diminishing its scariness in your mind.

"I want to lose 10 pounds- that's probably as tough as putting a man on the moon."

Imagine telling an iron man finisher how proud you are of your one-mile long workout this morning.

Ok! Whew! We got through it. The stock-take of your core personality traits. The stock-take of your drivers. I am hopeful, but also quite sure that you will have found a number of items that you need to pay attention to, and that if you did do a better job at, you would be able to exponentially increase your results, and open new doors of opportunity for yourself.

I want to leave you with the story of the red paperclip. The story goes that the person started with one red paperclip and traded it up 14 times. 14 trades later he had turned that red paperclip into a house. While I am not sure if the red paper clip is a true story, I am absolutely sure that people can trade up their old emotions and internals for new, higher yielding ones. We are going to do that very thing here internally. We are going to trade up and trade up until our internals pay us off with the life of our dreams.

"Sometimes you have to play a long time to learn to play like yourself"
--Miles Davis

CHAPTER 2: GOAL SETTING.

"A dream is just a dream. A goal is a dream with
a plan and a deadline."
—*Harvey Mackey*

A ccomplishments are based on actions, not on thoughts. But the thought always comes before the action. Achievement starts with an idea, a perspective, a point of view or even an attitude. However, it is only actions that can bring your masterpiece to life. At the end of the day, living your life can be thought of as a process of expressing your beliefs and desires through action.

At the very top of the food chain, you have Roger Federer being able to take the action of playing his best point of the day at the most important moment. On the most basic level, this is the reason why he makes the kind of money that he does, because when he takes a series of actions on a tennis court, like Tarzan swinging from vine to vine, he is able to swing to the proverbial other side of the swamp, while very seldomly falling into the crocodile infested pit. His actions lead to victory. I want you to start building the idea of your superstar day. A day where you eat right, call all the right people, hit the gym hard, help 10 little grannies cross the street. It's you…only, better!

That's why we are all here, we want our actions to lead to more victory. We want to become winners. Better yet, we want to become consistent winners. We want to overcome our demons, face our fears and come out shining on the other side. We want to find that magical state of performance that is not hindered by anger, or injury, or financial pressure, self-esteem, our deepest fears - we want to be able to FLY. In order to FLY, we are going to need wings. The first step to sprouting some wings is to have a plan and a map. A plan to make you extraordinary by design.

Bringing a great idea to life is orders of magnitude more difficult than just having a great idea. Having the idea is a great starting point, but the real art form comes with bringing the idea to life. Many a person has landed on the lush green island of a great idea, but few have survived the treacherous journey across the rickety bridge of execution.

Great goal setting seeks to unlock your true potential by building a road to express your higher inner core values and your best ideas. Whether you want to make the connection or not, you are EXPRESSING your values with each choice and action you make, for example:

- Choose to sleep in for another hour - you are expressing that you have the extra time available. Your goal for the day can wait.

- Choose to study biology - you are expressing you don't have enough liking for music to study it, or math, or sociology.

- Choose high paying job with low quality of life - you are saying money is more important than fun.

We are always EXPRESSING OUR VALUES. You can identify someone who values family, someone who values money, someone who values hard work, persistence, and so on. Where most people can go wrong is that they think about goal setting as the place where they decide to change the world, quadruple their earnings and write a Pulitzer Prize winning novel. They think of it as the place where they change the way humans live forever. Because their goals are so big, it's hard for their internal systems to believe, and therefore, they have a hard time gathering the necessary resources to get started, keep going, and stay the course. Early on in my life, I used to have a love/hate relationship with goal setting. I think one of the main reasons for this was that I used to write down a lot of OUTCOME based goals. Wanting to win Wimbledon is noble, and looks good on paper, but what really is necessary are the PROCESS goals.

Let's do just a little background on goals and go through the core points that you need to know. Then let's see if you can have a crack at putting together your preliminary goal list.

Step 1: Set up your goal categories.

Understand that really big goals will require you to dedicate yourself almost wholeheartedly to the one task, meaning that you forfeit time and achievement in other areas. And if this is that kind of a year for you, then more power to you! Outside of that, however, we need to balance our approach to goal setting, and even though this book is about your mental conditioning, it's important to break your life down into its major component pieces.

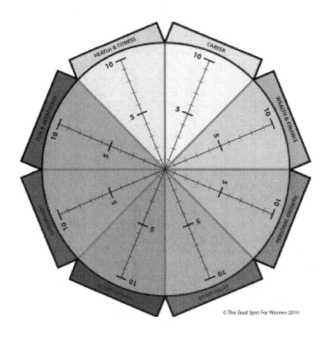

Health goals: A pretty obvious choice for the top of the list. It's hard to do stuff when you are sick, dying, or dead. Looking after your body and being on top of your health habits is key.

Career goals: Most of us take tremendous pride in our work and in our skillset. Work gives us the place to express a side of us that leads to many rewards both internally and externally. It is important to map out where you want to be in 5 to 10 years time. Sometimes we get stuck in a rut, and have not experienced career growth in a while, and now is the time to add to and build on that skill set.

Friend and family goals: We are all blessed with some really cool people to look after and hang with in this lifetime. Make sure to write down some goals that deal with making their experience on this planet that much sweeter!

Personal Development/Educational goals: That's the big piece of this book, we are working on developing your internal game, and shedding some bad habits in lieu of some major upgrades that allow you to crush all your other goals on this list!

Financial goals: Money is the lubricant of our lives. I don't know if I necessarily subscribe to the idea of making my life only about acquiring this lubricant, but without it, machines tend to break down and break down fast. Money is the tool that allows you to do the things you want and need to do in this world. It's really smart to have a good budget, and to have a plan for where you are heading financially. Also, saving and budgeting helps you to avoid spending on junk now, remembering that you want your cash for your epic trip coming up a few months from now.

Fun Goals: One of the absolute coolest things about having your game nice and tight and organized, is that your get to have fun and relax. I am a huge believer in the fact that you have one life, 80 years. Make the most of it. So you need to have some goals that are your fun category. Otherwise what's all this work for?

Step 2: What makes a good goal?

Probably not a bad idea to go through what makes a goal a good one. The key idea with a goal is quite simple. You are trying to be as logical and thoughtful about what you want to achieve over certain timeframes. There is a dreamy element to goal setting, no doubt, but if you want to really walk the walk, there are a ton of common-sense items that will be coming out onto your goal sheet.

S.M.A.R.T goals have been around for a while now, and it still stands as the best way to think about how to make your goals: **Specific, Measurable, Attainable, Relevant, Time bound.**

Specific.

You need to have an idea of what you are shooting for. Something like a "good" year is not really going to help you much because you need to be a more specific about what exactly a "good" year entails.

Measurable.

We want to be able to measure our success. Your goal has to have some type of built in accountability, a way of measuring if you are going forward or backwards, so that you can adjustment and course correct as needs be.

Attainable.

With regards to attainability, recognize that it's a sliding scale. Your long-term goals are maybe a little bit of a stretch, while your short term or day to day goals should be absolutely attainable with good management of your time for the day.

Relevant.

Relevance speaks to motivation. Some things might not be very motivating, like losing 10 pounds, but might be necessary for you to get the blood pressure down, so it's very relevant.

Time bound.

A lot of your goals will be a "best guess" situation. It might take a longer or shorter timeframe than you imagined, you might be ahead of schedule or falling behind. Filling in the "by when?" part of the goal is essential to actually doing it. You need to know how much work you need to do on a daily basis, weekly basis, and quarterly basis. Without this, there is simply too much doubt, indecision and lack of focus to be realistic about causing the outcomes you want in your life.

Slippage

You need to keep some mental room for slippage and failure. You will miss targets, you will miss deadlines and make mistakes. You will fall back into old habits. You will need a few restarts. You will regress.

I really want to make that point in order to actually get things completed, you need to understand this principle. What are you going to do when things go wrong? What are you going to do when the unforeseens hit? You need these to be a part of your goal-setting also. You need catastrophe goals. Take a minute and write down what you plan to do when the proverbial sh%$ hits the fan.

As much as it would be fun to be a robot and be able to act routinely without any hiccups, pauses or interferences, being a human means that you will always have to win the debate inside your own head and convince yourself to do stuff. Sometimes it can be something as simple as getting out of bed;

You: "Ok, time to get up now!"

Still you: "But it's so warm and comfy"

More you: "I'll make you a nice cup of coffee, and then we can chill for five minutes before the babies wake up…."

You again: "but it's so warm and comfy…!"

This inner dialogue never stops, and the reality is that sometimes we are going to lose the argument against ourselves. In order to build really long standing, really awesome habits, you are basically showing off how many times you were able to win the argument. When you see someone who is in the gym for his 80th session in a row, basically you are looking at a debate champion.

So have your arguments ready. Polish your responses, your rebuttals. Be ready for slippage to try and put its greasy little hands on you and conquer this beast one small victory at a time.

For anyone who has seen the movie, "A Beautiful Mind" the main character has delusions, living with three fictitious characters inside his head. Eventually he figures this out and decides to simply ignore them. They never go away, but he just chooses not to speak to them anymore. The gang of time thieves that live in your head, that try and cause you to slip, will never go away. You just get really good at paying no attention to them.

3 Types of Goals
Long Terms Goals

When we begin the Goal setting session, it is important to understand the big categories in our lives: Health, Work, Family, Finances, Personal Growth, and Experience. We want to write down the big picture for each one of these, the vision. Long term goals can be exhilarating to think about and can create a lot of emotion and positivity inside of us, but the practical reality of planning and managing the path to achieving your long term goal can be daunting. My guess is that if we were able to collect all of the goal sheets on which we have written down long term goals, we would find a whole lot of missed targets. I'll bet you would find a whole lot of astronauts that have turned into accountants, future Wimbledon champions (in my case) that have turned into Entrepreneurs.

It's hard to get some of the big, directional long-term goals right, but that doesn't mean we shouldn't make them. It just means we might have to course correct and sit down and make new goals more often.

Write down one decent goal for each category that's on your list. Since this book is focused on your internals and building your key internals and mental toughness-- we want to make that the focus point, and maybe choose other goals that support our quest to improve our mental strength and internal composition.

Medium Term Goals

As we bring the timelines in to the 6 months to 1-year range, we start being able to be a lot more accurate in our assumptions. We might not be spot on, but we should be in the ballpark a lot more than our 5 and 10-year goals.

If you do a good job, and experience only minor setbacks, you should reach certain checkpoints at the 3 month, 6 month and 1 year marker. These are the goals you should get excited about, these are the ones you are going to hit, or be right nearby.

An interesting story that is worth telling here. When you do 20 pushups, and you are starting to fail around number 17, the feeling of failure and burn kicks in. You shake and wobble, and finally you fall down around 21 or 22.

How does this feeling differ from someone who can do 40 pushups, and starts to feel the burn at number 37? Or 57? The answer is: **it doesn't.** You feel just as tired in either case, even though your tolerance or limit has increased. What this means is: It's always going to require effort and planning to hit your goals, whether they are about saving a few bucks, or starting a large multinational corporation.

Short term goals

These are your money makers. Most of the people I work with are decent at this skill set, because modern life is so demanding of your time. Without a day planner and calendar, most people would miss far too many important events. We have a head start. What we need to watch out for is having to do list items that get us through the day, but not having the to do list items that are designed to change our lives. In other words, we all know what we HAVE to do every week. We want to make sure to focus on and build goals for what we NEED to do in order to make progress in the areas we want to change and grow in.

I set a lot of short-term goals and almost always have my lists and phone to do app working, and I have made it a habit to do a thorough spring cleaning of the list every Sunday. I take 2 hours early in the morning, with my cup of coffee on the balcony, and go through what was done, what was not done, what I think needs to be done, and what can wait versus what needed to have happened yesterday.

71

Process.

A great exercise here is to actually take a minute to see yourself in the "superhero" lens. What would you do if you had unlimited energy, what does a really well lived day look like? Instead of playing Candy Crush, you call a buddy? Instead of watching a show in the lunchroom you fire off some pushups? Instead of hitting the vending machine, you whip out your steamed vegetables that you purposefully prepared the night before? You take a moment at lunch to tick off some items on your newly formed to do list habit?

Get creative! Imagine a really awesome day, well executed by you. Now write down the areas where you fall short. Planning? Need rest and space out time?

Lather. Rinse. Repeat.

No matter what- you have to get into the habit of going over your goals. Refining, modifying, adapting. You have to use your newly developed thick skin to accept your failures and look them in the eye as worthy adversaries. You need to get a nice big fat grin as you think of a new and even more awesome way to tackle the problem. You need to affirm yourself, give yourself some positive reinforcement.

Realistically, we spend the vast majority of time striving to achieve goals rather than actually achieving them, so you really need to enjoy the process. And realistically, the world does not stop when you do achieve a goal. We tend to celebrate briefly, and move on, so have some fun with it.

Think of it this way. As an athlete, you spend way more time preparing for competition that actually competing, so you have to get good at and enjoy the preparation part. It's going to take you a lot of checkboxes before you win Wimbledon or get the Pulitzer Prize.

Keep in mind we are almost all united in our quest to close the gap between our potential and the results we are actually achieving.

MEGA ULTRA TIP: If there is one habit you should build, and just one, it is to set a regular time to review your goals!

Once a week, set up a time, go through, check off the completed ones, make your new ones for the upcoming week.

REWARD TIME!

Find something that you love as a reward for your hard work. I remember as a kid we hit a rough spot, just after the 1988 stock market crash. We were devastated, financially ruined and ended up downgrading from a nice 3-bedroom house to a 700 square foot apartment. We didn't have 2 cents to rub together. I remember my mom going back to work and having to sit in the corridor of the night school, while she took her classes to finish her degree. It was hard times. We had some pretty powerful adjusting to do. I remember my Mom going for an interview- this was big- it was a great job and it was about to propel us back to being able to buy a couple of goodies. She promised us that she would take us out for a cup of coffee or tea- (we were still too poor to buy food at the restaurant) if she got the job.

I will never forget that cup of coffee. That felt like a million dollars. It crystallized something inside of me too. I realized that we are all trying to achieve, whether your goals are big or small, they are YOURS and that makes them special and worth chasing!

That REWARD also etched something in my mind, it created a trigger. That process, far from being destructive, ended up being one of the most important for my definition of who I was. I was going to play professional tennis anyway. I was going to go to an amazing Division 1 university. I was going to start my own companies. That one little cup of coffee, that moment of triumph against my darkest days, has seared forever in me a knowledge that it CAN be done.

So, even if the reward is small, take those five minutes to create that magical special moment where you reward yourself and reflect on the journey so far!

Addicted to mediocrity

When you are a smoker of cigarettes, you face the justification wall somewhere around 20 times per day. You get the craving, and suddenly you start thinking that it is time to find an opportunity to smoke. Then the inner dialogue starts: "Maybe we should skip this one. Maybe it's time to stop. I am kinda sick of this habit. Ok, well, let's have this one, and then let's make some decisions before the next one."

That insidious loop that we just witnessed is what a smoker goes through to justify his next cigarette.

This justification loop is not limited to smokers though. We all have it. Once you set up your goals, you are going to encounter it front and center, because you are going to have to justify reasons for not sticking to timelines, or not completing tasks, or not doing what you said you were going to. And just like the smoker reaches for his pack of cigarettes, you are going to be tempted to reach for your bad habit or reach for your act of mediocrity.

Remember this, when you work out, it takes just as much effort when you are fit as when you are unfit. Your heart rate pounding at 180 when you are unfit feels exactly the same as you heart rate pounding at 180 when you are fit. It only takes a little longer to get there.

Whether your actions for the day are legendary, or whether they are poor, you are still going to take actions. And since you can't escape having to take action, it might as well be good one.

Before we kick off our journey, take the time to write down all the reasons why you should act, why do you want to make some changes, why you can't wait to be on the road to living your day in an enhanced, better way.

Bucket list.

It's a hard question. What do you want from this life? Really want? Travel? Family? Career? For a lot of people, it's easy to get overwhelmed by the enormity of trying to spend your 80 years on something worthwhile, yet fun, yet challenging, but also inspiring.

What we do know as fact is that the clock is ticking, and those minutes are being spent, whether you are fully in control of the spending or not. With that being said, it makes sense to get a grip on that process, and YOU decide how you spend your time.

The bucket list is just a wonderful exercise. These could be called long term goals, but I don't consider them that, because they are not actually the "serious" part of building your life.

This is the dreamy part, where you imagine being able to do anything you wanted, uninhibited by work, or finances, or circumstance, and you write down some things that would just be absolutely awesome! A dream holiday, a 1 year sabbatical to travel the world. Just have fun with it. Be creative, stir up the juices.

WABI-SABI, BABY!

It makes sense to end off this section on goal setting with a Japanese idea. Wabi Sabi. At its core it refers to wisdom and natural simplicity, and perhaps more accurately, flawed beauty. Wabi-sabi nurtures all that is authentic by acknowledging three simple realities: nothing lasts, nothing is finished, and nothing is perfect. *Wabi* can also refer to quirks and anomalies arising from the process of construction, which add uniqueness and elegance to the object. *Sabi* is beauty or serenity that comes with age, when the life of the object and its impermanence are evidenced in its patina and wear, or in any visible repairs. We have referenced the idea of being a great artist in the game of life earlier in this book, and I want you to think about that now again as you finalize your road map and goal setting.

We are going to go after these goals with energy and vigor, put our souls on the line, give ourselves a chance to grow in directions we never thought we could. But, in the back of your mind, knowing that the little nicks and cuts, little quirks and slight imperfections from the attempt to create something of a masterpiece, are beautiful in their own right. We are going to own them and wear them proudly. Your unique viewpoint, your unique translation of the art that is your life, will be intrinsically gorgeous.

Accomplishments are based on actions, not on thoughts. But the thought always comes before the action. Achievement starts with an idea, a perspective, a point of view or even an attitude. However, it is only actions that can bring your masterpiece to life.

OK, grab your stack of goals, and let's move on to building the mothership compadre!!

CHAPTER 3: SELF AWARENESS

When I think of the idea of self-awareness, I often think of myself as a pimply faced teen walking up to a girl for the first time to ask her out. I know just how many breaths per minute I am taking, palms sweating profusely, worried to shake hands because then she will notice how sweaty my hands are, "Is my hair ok? Am I going to stutter? Oh god, this is going to be a disaster, and everyone at school is going to know about it…..!?"

Sounds about right, a complete emotional wreck, and getting to the words "Hi Sally" is about the same as being strapped to the bungee cord and actually jumping when the countdown gets to zero.

You have such a heightened sense of self awareness in that moment.

Contrast this to 20 years later. You open the door to grab a newspaper, it's 11:00 am on a Saturday, you are still in your robe. You open the door, waving at the neighbors. Your kids are going "DAD, please don't, oh GOD, Anders is going to see us, he is in my math class dad!!! NOOOOOO"

You are probably not self-aware enough… Or you are quite self-aware and just have a devilish sense of humor…

Self-awareness is a huge component to being successful. Think of the modern car, and the abundance of sensors that help you monitor your vehicle. Fuel sensor, temperature gauge, seat belt sensor, airbags, engine temperature, only to name a few. Sometimes we don't even realize how important that sensor is until we don't have it anymore. Imagine for example, if your fuel sensor breaks down. Now you don't know how much fuel you have left. You have to guess, and of course to be safe, you end up carrying a can of gas in the back of your car or stopping at the gas station more frequently.

This can also go the other way. You can have a sensor that gives a false positive. I happened to own a BMW and the passenger side seatbelt alarm was defective. For no reason it would start to *ding ding*, giving the alarm that the seatbelt was not plugged in, even though there was no person in the seat. The sound of course is designed to penetrate deep into your soul and the involuntary clenching it causes has been known to chip teeth. So you pull over and make sure that you click the seatbelt in.

We have the mental sensors going off all the time. For some people, it's the, "let's get mad now" sensor, and before they know it, they are yelling or punching a wall.

For some people it's the, "let's start doubting ourselves now" sensor, and just as they start to build some momentum, they self- sabotage because of this faulty sensor.

For some people it's the "let's panic now" sensor- as panic, agitation, restlessness set in.

There is the "I need gratification now" sensor.

For all of us, we have to examine what sets off our sensors. Each emotion is extremely well designed and has a very necessary function in ensuring that we navigate through life well. But, our sensors can become muddled, and they can trigger at the wrong time.

What's important for us as we work on building ourselves up, is to develop a sensory system that is able to help us navigate towards our goals. We need to have a little voice inside our head that is able to direct and guide us in as straight a line as possible to the next progressionary step on the path towards achievement of a goal. When well built, we have a system that is able to generate good ideas into our head repeatedly. When I was playing my best tennis, I could rely on my ideas and trust their accuracy. I did not have to second guess. You could say that when you are playing well, you can trust your instincts. Developing good instincts takes time, practice, and a good relationship with yourself. With practice, your inner voice becomes a mega-sensor, steering you through the inertia, the doubt, and any other goal eating internals. Wouldn't it be nice is the following example was how your inner voice sounded:

"Choose the vegetable over the fried food"

"Let's get to bed early- and be fresh for tomorrow"

"Let's get up early and write down those good ideas before we forget them"

Well developed, it's a lot like having a good life coach inside your head. And once you and the voice inside your head have become good friends and you have a trust that the thoughts and ideas produced by your brain to guide you have good direction, then you really can be especially effective.

If it's the other way around, and the voice inside your head is giving poor feedback, then you are going to miss opportunities. You are going to sleep in, you are going to eat the donut, and you are going to skip out on putting the work into the responsibilities that are good for you.

A good knowledge of your value system, your 9 core internal categories from the previous chapter, and a well-developed sensory system to monitor the implementation of the actions necessary to complete the various steps, is going to go a long way towards turning you into a goal munching machine.

Are your cells influenced by thought?

Does the mind have control over what the body is doing? By thinking certain thoughts, can you become more alert, more aware? By denying yourself certain thoughts, can you switch off parts of yourself that are ineffective. Can you practice the art of switching on and off various parts of your thinking system, and develop this as an art that allows you fluidity as a person, capable of flexible growth and adaptation? If you have a negative outlook, can it lead to depression of your immune system, can it lead to diminished response from your senses? If yes, then you most likely won't process information well! It is imperative that you know what it is you need to pay attention to. You need to be able to identify and think "I am doing it again." Once you learn to identify the behavior, when it is happening, you finally have a chance to do something about it.

I think the story of Martin Strel, the marathon swimmer who has swum almost all the rivers in the world. He has completed the Danube, Mississippi, Parana, Yangtze, and finally the Amazon river. Yes. That's over 10,000 miles of swimming. He talks about when he set off and he had so much doubt, he was so focused on every stroke, counting 1,2,3,4,5... It was agonizing, slow, painful, and he had no idea of how he was actually going to do it. He pushed. He struggled on. And then, on the Danube, he had a breakthrough.

In his own words:

" I wasn't so confident at the beginning. I was very afraid. I didn't sleep. My pulse was very high, even in the Amazon. On the Amazon was a terrible moment, I was attacked by piranhas. Your back, you feel fire. They eat so fast. It is still the longest swim in history."

"On the Mississippi, I was touched by lightning. I was unconscious one minute. It pushed me out of the water, I was flying like a plane. I stopped for a couple of minutes. Then, GO Martin GO!

"Most of the people don't understand how you can swim 12 hours per day. When I swim, it is impossible to think about the stoke under the water. I even used to count these, one, two, three, four, five…. In the beginning, that was terrible. It was lots of pain. Swimming hours and hours in the oceans, lakes, rivers. Many times, I said to myself, 'It's simply too hard' You have tears in the eyes, you don't know how to move this, what to do, but you have to swim, you have to finish this. It was so hard to swim."

" And then, on the Danube…. It happened. I FOUND A WAY. It is hard for me to explain what is, meditation or hypnotization. Here is something what helps me a lot. It happened while I was swimming. My concentration is very, very deep like meditation. And then, when it is done. I don't feel pain anymore. Can somebody explain it to me, something? Some physician, scientist could say, 'that is not possible' Sure. For him it is not possible, but

it's possible for me. I think that everything is here in your brain, here."

-Martin Strel.

It is so incredibly hard to believe that what you are about to embark on actually has a chance of coming true. It is so hard to BELIEVE in yourself, your ideas. It is so hard to BELIEVE that you will go beyond the obstacles, that your resolve will hold. It's hard to even imagine the exact moment when you will become a non-smoker. It's hard to imagine that you will find love again. It's hard to imagine you will keep your new healthy habits, get the promotion, settle into your new career. Martin Strel's story has already happened to you, in its own way. Perhaps you had a tough break up somewhere along the way? Do you remember the exact moment when the pain stopped? When you were ready to move on? What about a tough math class, you thought you would never get through? Do you remember the exact moment when you understood calculus?

You just never know the moment when you will have your breakthroughs. But you will. And on the other side of these breakthroughs lies an unimaginable world of possibilities. The capacity to swim the world's longest rivers, set world records, and achieve the ideas your vision is able to create. I want you to reimagine your life story. Imagine for a moment that not all the chapters have been written yet. You can erase the chapters you don't like, rewrite them in a far better way.

Find YOUR WAY.

How do you improve self-awareness?

Engineering any sensor requires knowing what it is you are trying to monitor. Building a fuel sensor will be different than building an air pressure sensor, and they both serve a different function. We all have a number of beliefs and internals that cause us to act or avoid action in our subconscious mind. Think of this like the apps running in the background of your cell phone. They are chewing memory, wasting resources, slowing down your phone. From time to time, you just need to hit the "check for apps running in the background" button.

Building the right loop between spending some time on going through your internal tool kit, which is what chapter 2 is all about, and then forming rock solid goals is a major step in creating the direction and action item that you now need to monitor.

With those two completed, you need to have your checkpoints, and you need to raise your state of awareness.

Remember that it is much easier for your body to revert back to old ways than it is to forge new ones, so you will certainly have to work your way through drag.

Here is my list for improving your self-awareness:

Observe yourself:

While you go through your day, you pay attention to the thoughts, ideas, inhibitions, frustrations that occur inside you in your different interactions.

Introspection:

This is where you think about what you have observed. Your objective is to try and understand the root and the "why?" behind certain behaviors.

Shift paradigm:

This is where you use powerful thoughts to overcome instinctive behaviors, and old stale habits. Understanding which thoughts or patterns no longer offer you any value.

Recalibration:

Take the time to ask yourself what it is that you want from this life. Ask yourself what you need to let go of. Ask yourself what you need to incorporate.

Engage:

Get out there and take action. All the while practicing being self-aware.

Ritual:

Athletes do this. Think about Rafael Nadal, how he compulsively moves his water bottles around to the exact perfect place. What he is actually doing is practicing one of his rituals. Find a cool, fun way to add 1 or two small rituals that shake you back to being self-aware.

BEWARE THE DENIAL TRAIN

My final suggestion in this chapter deals with the mental trick "check-mate". You have to be aware of one of the more powerful human emotions that is at work before you can really get off the ground. We tend to smooth over the rough ideas in our mind, a tendency to gloss over the more graphic details with gloriously crafted euphemisms.

In short, we tend to say things are going along just swell even when they are not. Part of it is the embarrassment of our friends finding out that we have any imperfections. The biggest part is simply acknowledgement of the fact that we need to make some changes. Why? Because the minute you actually stand up and say: "I gotta work on my self-esteem," and you admit that the beast is real, then you feel compelled, you actually have to do something about it.

For a lot of us, that is the scariest part of all. Realizing that things are actually not on track. Realizing that you have been in a hypnotic, zombie like state, on some escalator to a nowhere land.

Waking up, jumping in. That's what taking your future by the kahuna's is about. That's what taking this giant canvas that is your life, grabbing the internals that are your paintbrush, and painting your masterpiece is all about!

Every child is an artist. The trouble is staying an artist when we grow up.

-Pablo Picasso.

Chapter 4: Habits

Raising your action level into the "difference making" category.

Once you get yourself motivated and figure out your game plan, the only logical next step is to take action. Enough action that it's ACTUALLY going to make a difference. If you can get your new actions to the point where you really are going to make a lasting impact, then you can expect to experience change. Once you have the actions that are going to make lasting, noticeable and legendary change, then we need to make these new actions permanent. *"Action Permanence" is the coup de grace of habit formation.*

Being able to develop and maintain a habit(s), as well as disassemble ones that are no longer useful to us, is a critical skill to develop. We are going to go into the trenches, taking grenades to develop a full understanding of where our habits come from, why the human brain relies on them so much, and how they can be both a hindrance or the key that unlocks your potential. We want to keep adding essential practices until your new patterns become second nature - the ground rules of how you operate. Habits can be like plants. As any good gardener will tell you, it takes the right environment, the correct homeostasis, to grow seedlings into full-fledged thriving plants. When you plant a habit, we want it to grow into Audrey 2 from the film Little Shop of Horrors.

There will be real obstacles that threaten to dislodge your new habits just as they start to sink their teeth into your life.

There will be unwanted habits that hang in there even though you have called in the mediums and had a seance to remove them. There will also be the slow and stealthy drip-drip-drip time wasting activities. Normal, everyday activities that end up taking most of your day and leave you with little time to build your remarkable new future. They are like ninjas that sneak into your house silently and sneak out unnoticed with a solid chunk of your precious time under their arms. You will have to develop and grow an understanding of how your world view and **perspective** influences your habits. For example, if you're coming from the point of view that you will do it tomorrow, that you have plenty of time, that you are actually just fine, you are going to cave in to the craftiest habit poison of all time- **justifications.**

The habit of finishing

We all know our GOAL actually can be achieved. Lose ten pounds, get the promotion, learn the new skill, pay off the house quicker. The goals that most of us think about are ACHIEVABLE. We don't need some self-help guru to make us CHANT them as a mantra twelve times per day to get to the point that we know they are achievable. We know because we are intelligent adults. We know we can achieve because we are surrounded by goals being achieved and success stories on a daily basis. We see people achieving goals just like ours all the time. We see Apple with the iPhone, Elon Musk's Tesla, and the U.A.E's development of stunning architectural marvels and feats of engineering. On a personal scale, we have also been witness to, and involved with, our own versions of systems that have worked, be it graduating from college, earning an MBA or Doctorate, starting our own companies. We are almost all successful and have good habits in one or more of our 9 cores. We understand success.

Our goal with this chapter is to build a knowledge of how habits work, what can break them, how you maintain them, and how to choose the right ones. Through the early part of this book, you built a list of goals and priorities, items that you need to complete in order to start bringing about real, measurable change. If you were to ever be walking along the beach and spot a shiny lamp glinting at you, only to rub it and activate the genie, one of your wishes would surely be, "teach me how to stay motivated, stay consistent and make it to the finish line."

What is the secret of the people who are able to finish stuff? Where can we get some of what *they* have? Our goals are right here, right in front of us. Achievable. If only we could just FINISH stuff. How easy is it to come home and just be too tired to do the workout? How easy is it to forget to plan and prepare the meals? How easy is it for work to be the excuse that stops you from achieving your personal goals? How easy is it to start having great fun with your babies and feel guilty to leave them and go do what you need to do? Life makes us tired. It's hard to balance family, work, personal growth, having fun, and reaching for the stars. We all know this. We all have a real danger of falling into a humdrum, survival mode, 5 out of 10, pattern. Doing just enough to get by.

What we need to do is build out the protocols. The sequence of actions that make everything possible. Success in any category, in any field, in anything that you dare to dream of, can only come about through consistent action. And in order to take consistent action, you have to build a pathway to taking that action as often as it is needed. This means it needs to fit in with your already busy schedule. This means you need to let go of other actions you quite enjoy. This means CHANGE.

We so often make the mistake of thinking that something needs to happen in order to kick off the conversion of your dreams to reality. We need the lucky break. The knock on the door from fate. Something external. The reality is we work from the inside out. We build a super-fit mind. This mind creates great ideas. Those ideas are actionable. This mind has the endurance to keep taking the right action. This mind is excited by challenges and does not run away and bury the dream in the sand like a dog-bone.

What we did in the first part of this book helped us to create a vision of what to strive for as a person. It helped us to clear conflicting ideas, so that we are not torn between which ideas to pour energy into. It helped us create clarity.

In order to be consistent, and to continuously achieve, we need to maintain this clarity. We need to remain objective in our choices, and consistently be able to determine which actions to pursue, and which ones to let go. In order to really conquer the world of habits, we need to build up our knowledge base. Let's science this bad boy a little bit, and take a look at:

Why habits form in the first place?

On a basic level, maybe it is a fun exercise to try and understand why habits evolved in the first place. If you consider that everything revolves around energy, and how much effort it takes to hunt food, eat it and process it, it stands to reason that our brain would look for shortcuts. Forming a habit is a great way of making a task automated, sort of like breathing and walking. We then have the freedom to use our saved energy to think of even better ways of hunting, fishing or using that energy.

PERCEPTION CAN BE KEY TO UNLOCKING NEW BEHAVIOURS.

One of the key things we now know about changing habits is that a _**shift in perception**_ can trigger a chain reaction of change that eventually radiates into all avenues of one's life. Recent research has shown that when they process an MRI scan on the brain of someone who has undergone major habit changes, they can still see the old neural pathways, but can also clearly see brand new neural pathways that "override" the old ones. As your habits change, so does your brain. They notice the areas of the brain where specific impulses are. Specific impulse areas light up when triggers occur, like when someone who is a smoker or ex-smoker sees a cigarette and that original craving sends the brain a message, "Oh! I want one!" Yet, we can simultaneously see a brand-new area where self-inhibition and self-discipline reside light up in the person with new habits. We now have come to know the phenomenon of a changing brain as neuroplasticity. This remarkable phenomenon means the brain is capable of change and can alter itself, dependent on the habits we form and enforce. This means that we have the power, through external actions to create lasting, permanent change to the structure of our own brains.

NEUROPLASTICITY IS THE WAY TO A NEW YOU.

Keep this in mind as you begin to make changes. The first steps are the hardest, your brain has the least new pathways to work with. As you develop and build a whole new brain wiring, it will become easier. It's not just individuals who are capable of shifting their habits. Companies can have massive transformations just from changing a few habits. We see a whole new wave of emphasis around corporate culture- how work gets done, interpersonal communication, and behavior toward the consumer.

Let's take a look at where habits can be extraordinarily useful:

- Habits can be extremely useful when you are exhausted and overwhelmed- and you need to make decisions. It might be much better to train yourself to automate each decision at the level of habit in those situations.

- Routines and habits can make it easier to work alongside people you can't stand

- Well-built triggers can cause long lasting positive spirals

- There might be very little you can't do if you get the habits right!

We all remember the old iPhone 3g commercial:
"There's an app for that".

Well, anything cool that's ever been done:
"There is a habit for that!".

THE INNER MECHANISMS OF HABITS

Research has been unlocking the key to habits and habit formation for years, with a much deeper understanding of how habits work coming as technology to probe the brain has improved. What we have recently discovered is that if you strap on a scanner capable of measuring activity in the brain and you give someone a new task to do, you will see a flurry of brain activity. When you repeat the task a couple of hundred times, you see a decrease in brain activity. This means that at first you need to CHOOSE what part of the movement to do when. The part of your brain than controls choices lights up. After a while, this choice becomes unconscious and the brain activity associated with decision making goes quiet. Believe it or not, even the brain activity associated with memory will go quiet.

The body relies on the basal ganglia, which is central to pattern development. In other words- these actions are not memorized, they are stored in the subconscious pattern area of the brain. Why does a super experienced pro have such a big advantage over you? Because he does not actually have to think in the highest-pressure situations- he is using pattern recognition. If you are new to it- your brain will be lighting up like a Christmas tree!!

LET'S BREAK IT DOWN LIKE A FRACTION. HOW DO HABITS WORK?

HABITS ARE BUILT ON A TRIGGER SYSTEM:

CUE-----> ROUTINE-----> REWARD

CUE: Trigger or signal that has been trained into the system to signal the beginning of a process.

ROUTINE: The actual process that begins once the cue has been received. Often times on automatic, once the cue has been received, the body will begin the activity often in a reactive way.

REWARD: Release of endorphins, calming effect, or other reward for completing the task.

Once you have a strongly developed cue, routine and reward structure, you begin to have feelings of anticipation, or cravings.

One of the key items to remember here is that once a habit is formed-- the brain stops fully participating in decision making. This means that unless you actively find new routines, the pattern will unfold automatically.

For our purposes, we need to capitalize on three very important points:

1. You can make your most important and most powerful success-oriented patterns into a habit.

2. You can FORCE bad tendencies into the background-ignoring the old bad tendencies can become just as easy as reaching for the cigarette used to be.

3. And, most importantly, it is possible to really key POWERFUL habits. Habits that seek to reach deep

into our potential and unlock the person we were meant to be.

Here is a big question. How do we shine the spotlight on our habits? If we have numerous ones that are operating on an unconscious level- and we are forming some new ones based on triggers that we might not be aware of- does this leave us in need of some habit "spring cleaning" from time to time? One of the most important tools in habit forming is CRAVINGS--- This is what makes cues and rewards work. One of the most obvious ones that we all have is toothpaste. That fizzy-bubbly sparkly feeling in your mouth is something we all look forward to everyday. But-- it was not always so. Most **toothpastes** contain Sodium Lauryl Sulfate which is a chemical used in **toothpaste** to create the **foaming** action. That combined with the delicious minty flavor equals an unmistakable CUE- ROUTINE-REWARD system. Try it. Go and buy a mint-less foamless toothpaste and see how miserable you are. It would lead to a binge session of Dr. Phil, it would render you utterly broken.

Let's take another look at the habit loop-- cue-routine-reward. A big problem with keeping your successful habits is that often the ROUTINE part of the equation is HARD WORK, and the REWARD part is years, maybe decades away. It becomes difficult to hang onto those habits for long enough to get the big reward one day...

It's also quite difficult to course correct. Because the feedback from what you are doing is not immediate, it's difficult to understand when to alter or modify the habit. With a sport, where failure is your reward for poor choices and habits, it's much easier to course correct- seeking a favorable result. With eating burgers, you don't feel the heart attack immediately, therefore it's possible to eat hamburgers for many years before finally getting the negative result.

THE REWARD CYCLE

The final piece in the loop is to give yourself a clear reward for completing the routine-- if you give yourself a beer, a show that you like, fishing trip on the weekend for sticking to your habits, you have a much better chance of keeping the habit. This is key element is completing the loop. Make sure to plan in the reward.

We can really manipulate the anticipation of the reward- if you have trained the habit system long enough   cue-------routine------reward, you start to see the spike in brain activity that says "I got a reward" happening before the actual reward is given or achieved.

What this means is that the cue now becomes a trigger for pleasure inside the brain.

DELAYED REWARD OR NO REWARD

When you start to anticipate a reward, but then don't receive it, a cycle of craving, frustration and acting out is created. We now have a new pattern:

CUE--HAPPINESS--- DELAYED REWARD-----FRUSTRATION---ANGER--AGITATION

Habits are so powerful because they create neurological cravings. Particularly strong habits can create obsessive behaviors. These can power through the strongest of disincentives, losing your job, family, house, income. Of course, we have some interim rewards that are extremely valuable. When we work hard, we get a sense of satisfaction which is extremely important! We also get endorphins after a tough workout. You get a sense of triumph from tracking your performances/growth. You win tournaments and titles/ prestige/ recognition.

If you want to build a habit, it is essential that you build a simple cue-- something that acts as the trigger. Then keep going long enough for your brain to start craving one of the rewards above. You might find for example that you have done well and are on track for 6 months or even a year of something, but then the habits break down because the stress of everyday life intervenes, and the habit loop is broken.

It is important is to be able to control how motivated you are. We all know that feeling when you have just fallen in love and you have a date that Friday evening. It's only Wednesday 10:00 a.m. but work feels like a breeze, you are floating on clouds and all the hard stuff actually feels like it's happening in an extremely easy way for now. This is what it can feel like when you are highly motivated.

What generally tends to happen, is that after you have been dating for a while, somewhere around 6 months into a normal routine, you cannot generate the same amount of emotion and happy feelings as you did in the very beginning for that situation. As a result, your behaviors change. You are not as motivated to go and buy flowers, not as motivated to open the door and not as motivated to buy and write those little special "I love you" cards. Many relationships end up paying the price as the habit changes that occur when you start dating are too different to the ones that form when everything "settles". What used to be patience and the ability to listen to your loved one's point of view, becomes intolerance, impatience.

ONE GALVANISING HABIT

Think about the one galvanizing habit- the idea would be that instead of focusing on winning more, you focus on becoming much more consistent. What does this mean though? In order to be genuinely consistent, able to be competitive in that department with some of the best in the world, you would need the following:

- More reading skills to see and react to opponents' shots

- More speed balance and agility on your own execution

- Much deeper tactical understanding to place balls outside danger zone, limit opponent's opportunity to shorten point.

- Increased mental capacity to concentrate more, deal with problems better and find solutions to problems faster

- Increased endurance.

This "one" change ends up having an enormous impact on so many of your other habit and forces change throughout the organism as a whole. We would describe this as a galvanizing habit because of the power that it has to "overhaul."

MIND BODY LINK

The mind and the body are inextricably linked. Human beings have the unique ability to imagine and recreate events in our minds, but what's interesting is that our bodies react to the imagined event showing measurable physiological changes.

This is the reason visualization is so powerful as a success tool. Once you get good at it, you can create the feelings and emotions of the situation as if it was real in your mind. This can help you to deal with those feelings way ahead of time, and so when you actually are in the situation, you are rehearsed, and accustomed to the atmosphere.

The converse is also true, and you can spend excessive time reliving negative past experiences and shaping your emotions based on pictures or images in your head that are not real. Let's take a look at how something like that might work. We will pick an action that you may have failed at before, like going up onto the dance floor and asking someone to dance.

You: "That girl/guy seems nice, let's go and ask them to dance, let's have some fun."

Inner you: "What if they say no?"

More inner you: "That will be so embarrassing, everyone will see you being rejected"

More inner you: "What if she says yes, your dance skills are atrocious. You look like a mountain goat licking salt off a cliff when you are out on the dance floor!"

You: "Yikes, this could end up being the worst experience of my life, worse than death… because I will have to live with the memory of this for the rest of my life!"

Well done you. You just made something pretty simple into a trauma that would require many years to recover from. And, it all happened in your head. This is a classic example of runaway negative visualization. You imagined the entire scenario in your head and played it out as if it was real, building up even more anxiety about the situation for next time. Only…. It never actually happened.

Let's take a look at the idea of pressure. As a tennis player, this is a concept that we run into almost every time we compete. Pressure is also to a large extent an imaginary concept. We start to make decisions and choices about the gravity or impetus of a situation.

Real You: "This is a huge situation."

Inner you: "This could change your life."

More inner you: "I hope you don't choke today."

You again: "you have been training your whole life for today, this means everything."

Well done, you have turned it into a life or death situation in your mind. Let's have a look at what physiological changes you have induced in your body as a result of your thinking:

These are the common feelings associated with pressure?

- Butterflies in the stomach

- Sweaty palms

- Tense muscles

- Nausea

- Lethargy

- Hyperactivity and restlessness

Keep in mind that nature has evolved us to have all of these symptoms as a way of helping us out. You get the same feelings your ancestors got when they stumbled upon a hungry lion. The only difference is you are competing for a trophy or doing a presentation for a big client. What makes this troublesome for us, is that the body is now having reactions as we prepare to complete the same habit that we always do. We are not just dealing with having to make our mind go quiet, the whole system is wired to respond right before we take action, and so when you want to break a habit, you will have to override your whole body as well as your mind.

YOUR HABITS: FOR SALE

Perhaps it might make you a little cautious too. Have you ever wondered if there is anyone out there who might have a vested interest in you forming certain habits? It might be worth a few million dollars or so to any company who can make you go and buy their product out of habit get you hooked on certain cues and then form a routine of using a product to get a reward.

I think we should take a second to talk about the advertising industry and their remarkable ability to influence and change people's habits. (Find examples here)

It's extremely interesting that we are unable to change our own habits sometimes, yet an outside source is successfully acting upon your habits and decision making with the goal of turning your CUE- ROUTINE-REWARD system into big dollars for them. If they have figured out how to create behaviors in you, then you can bet your bottom dollar that it is critical that you understand and can build and destroy your own habits as you see fit. Stay out of my basal ganglia dudes!!

YOU MIGHT HAVE TO DIE IN ORDER TO TRULY LIVE. THE IDENTITY LINK

Have you ever wondered how it was possible for someone to make drastic changes? We all know someone who was heading down the road to nowhere, and who seemed compelled to continue making the choices that would keep them trapped on that road. To me it was always easier to understand from the point of view of a successful person who had encountered a breakdown, someone who had been there before, and had maybe had a meltdown. They then got "over it" and got back on track. But seeing someone go from a super low base and have a personality transplant, now this is fascinating. Interesting, because of course we have our identity, a way in which we see ourselves. We associate our thinking, our beliefs, our actions, and our results with our personality. This is who we are. Right?

We see two starkly different outcomes. The first is a mind that locks onto a personality type and becomes rigidly attached. Think of the cult or indoctrinated mind. This mind has taken on an identity that has been handed to them and can hardly function without this transplanted identity. This mind has had trouble forming its own identity, and as a result is very vulnerable. There are people who get trapped in an identity for years, believing that this situation is "their destiny", and even when they have every good reason to change, they don't.

Then, in stark contrast, are people who have a concept of "who they are" that is very fluid, they're seemingly able to adjust and let go of things quite easily. I have seen people who are the victims of crimes that could most certainly define them, instead choose to be defined in a completely different way. They are able to hold onto their core beliefs, and their set of boundaries, but they have the flexibility to use those across a number of environments and skill sets. If there is one thing that we can extrapolate from all of this, it is that we just simply are not who we believe we are. It is a necessary function of the brain to build up a self-image, but it has been proven over and over again that if you change the circumstances, put one twin in Kazakhstan and the other in the USA, you are going to end up with very different people. Change your inner chemistry, your beliefs, your triggers, your action list, your self-perception, and you are going to experience a results transplant, it's that simple. There are very few things we cannot change about our personality. These concrete, cold, hard fact lead us to some very simple questions:

Why settle for a you that is way less than you can be?

Why accept habits into your life that are not helpful?

THE HABIT BREAKERS
THE DELUSIONS

The addict delusion:

"I can start anytime I want to- I could easily be a marathon runner if I wanted to be- I just don't really want to" is a big part of the problem, we all have this delusion that it's easier than it actually is- and it's only when we actually get going that we realize how tough it's going to be.

I need my big break delusion:

What would happen if Bill Gates decided to hand Microsoft over to me? Where would it be in 5 years? My guess is: IN DEEP TROUBLE. Why? Because I know absolutely nothing about a giant computer software business- and my decisions would almost undoubtedly be based on poor information and poor habits with regard to that industry.

My ideas are my own delusion:

Habit forming can happen at an ideological level- People can become addicted to acts of terror. People can make a habit out of conflict. They can make a habit of supporting a regime. Most importantly they make habits out of lots of responses to situations, responses to challenges, responses to people, and many of the day to day items that slowly build your life.

I am not affected by my culture delusion:

People think they are separate from their cultures, and the cities and villages they live in. They believe that has not affected their belief system and the way they form decisions and self-opinion.

I know what's good for me delusion:

The metaphor here is someone who has been overeating or who has poor eating habits. Your body lacks nutrients and thus tells you it's still hungry. The food you are eating is not meeting your bodies requirements for the day. You get stuck in a cycle where you eat, but don't satisfy, then eat more, but still have cravings.

This same cycle can happen in your emotional core. Your sensory system is telling you that you need to make some changes, but unfortunately the things you reach for to satisfy those emotional cravings, end up being devoid of emotional nutrients, and so no matter how many times you are hungry for them, they don't fill you up.

SELF SABOTAGE

We have done the work of reconnecting with our goals, our true inner values. We have interrupted ingrained patterns of thought and action and have strengthened deliberation and self-regulation processes. We are on the road. New habits are in place, and all that's left now is to stay on the road.

Now we have to look out for one of the most insidious little habit breakers, self-sabotage. Behavior is said to be self-sabotaging when it creates problems and interferes with long-standing goals.

Examples: You have a great meeting with someone- only to not call them back to close the deal.

You have a great workout week, only to blow out 5000 calories per day on the weekend.

You are doing well with saving some cash, only to blow it all on one purse randomly.

Self-sabotage is caused by a number of things, but here are the most common ones

Not worthy: Deep down you don't have the confidence that you deserve better and are actually terrified of what the new you will act and feel like. Self-sabotage is a desperate attempt to hold on to a more known, more comfortable you.

People like to be consistent — our actions tend to be in sync with our beliefs and values. When they aren't, we try to line them up again. If we start to rack up the victories and accomplishments, yet still view ourselves as flawed, worthless, incapable, or deficient, we pull the plug to get rid of the growing distance between these two ideas, our results and our values. If it feels bad to fail, it actually feels even worse to succeed. There is even a name for this in the psychology annals, it's called: Imposter syndrome.

Control: People can be addicted to control. Unknowns can blindside you. Self-sabotage can be a twisted way of keeping control. You control the downside, rather than having it be something unknown that surprises you and brings you down.

Early Failure acceptance: Failure is awful. It's as powerful a motivator as there can be for the human mind. For some people, it's more palatable to start the failure process and experience the feelings of their idea not working out now, rather than be all excited and actually have hope, only to fail and have to deal with it then. Self-sabotage can be a reaction to the fear of failure.

Pressure and trust: "It was a big moment, everything was on the line, that's why I went back to what I knew. That's why I changed back to my old habit."

What this person is really saying is that they trusted the system most of the time, but in the biggest moments, they did not, their belief in it broke down. This is why they felt like they had to do something different when it really mattered.

Culture and group habits. Being around the wrong people can be a major habit breaker. The research states that the closest five people to you define who you are. If you join the Crips or the Bloods, chances are you are going to have some hindrance getting to Harvard!

Your inner fitness, the strength and stamina of your mind at any given moment is something we really need to consider here. You can be physically fit regardless of socio-economic background. It's the great equalizer. That gym weight feels the same to the guy who lives in a one bedroom as it does to the guy with the built-in helicopter landing pad in his house. Keep this in mind as you are building yourself. Life is not about the resources you start with. Great thoughts which lead to great actions are the great equalizer. The reason so many people from all walks of life have done brilliant things, is because they have been able to create fantastic ideas. You need to be in the Habit of thinking. Thinking big. Using your imagination. Actioning your ideas. Expressing your vision. This is the truly great equalizer in life.

So many people are in the excuse business. They prefer to conjure up reasons why things have not worked out. For those who want to be successful, your brain

CHAPTER 5: THE PROCESS

Building habits is a fundamental step in successfully doing anything at all. But that is only half the battle. Once you have built up a capacity to show up and be there performing your chosen task, the next question becomes one of HOW you are performing that task. Getting yourself up and out of bed and into the gym is an excellent start, but the hard part is delivering an excellent, hard hitting, high impact workout.

We generally have a process for just about everything, from what we like to wear, to what we like to eat, what we like to think about and what we like to talk about. What makes us angry, what makes us switch off, and what makes us break our commitments to ourselves. We have generally evolved our method and process over the years, some of the items have been handed down to us from parents or family members, and some have been picked up along the way.

As far as our main goal, we are trying to find and establish new processes that are very well aligned with our new goals and constructively support achievement. What this means is that we are going to need to take control over a number of key processes in our lives and become a process driven person. The prevailing logic here is that given the choice to become an instant millionaire by stealing from a little old granny, or staying poor a little while longer while implementing a thoughtful, consistent methodology, we can trust that our choice of actions are so well built that we can quite easily choose the latter, knowing that success is an inevitable byproduct of the process we have built.

PROCESS DRIVEN PROBLEM SOLVING:

Here we are trying to develop a formal process as your main go-to when confronted with a problem. Process driven problem solving has some big advantages, most notably, when you are confronted with a problem, you can sidestep freaking out as you know you have a formal method of looking at the problem and creating an action plan. You can either follow a proven system that has worked in the past or use a process driven approach to building a new solution on the fly.

Here is an example of a process driven approach to problem solving:

1. Describe and understand the problem

2. Make an inventory of resources available to solve problem

3. Research and find expert opinions to guide decision making process

4. Make decision and make it actionable

5. Observe results, adjust and improvise

By clearly defining the steps in your procedure, it is easy to modify, adjust and improve over the years, which means that as you evolve and face more obstacles, you end up with a master-level ability to deconstruct and answer life's most challenging questions.

PROCESS DRIVEN EMOTIONAL CONTROL:

One of the most important elements for competing well as a professional "life-player" is having control over your emotions. Fear, uncertainty, panic, hope, and the myriad of others that are all firing and triggering in your head can make it extremely noisy in there. This noise can make it very difficult to create a decent output to the stimulus or input you are receiving. You need to understand which internal states suit you best and are ideal for your top performance.

Understanding how much fear you can constructively deal with, and how much anxiety, confusion you can have in your environment and still thrive is critical. Understanding how you cope, when to trigger coping mechanisms, and how to calm or amp yourself up are all very important. Understand when your ego is kicking in.

Finally, arguably the most important concept you can master as far as emotions go is how to MANUFACTURE emotions on demand. I think of the emerging technology of 3D printers, and what this means for efficiency world-wide. Now you don't have to search on Google to find your car part in Lithuania, try to bargain with the person using Google translate and have the part sent only to arrive 3 weeks later. All the while having to Uber it while you wait to repair your car. Too inefficient.

Now, you can look up the part, and have it manufactured right at home. Click, choose done. Much more efficient. The best emotional players in the game of life are able to do this. They don't mess around with waiting for three weeks to get motivated, to get hungry, to get action based. They can manufacture these emotions on demand. They can override their instinctive feelings and build the correct and necessary ones quickly. Think of the freedom and power you will unlock if you are able to manufacture necessary emotions, all on demand?

PROCESS FOR FINDING THE RIGHT EXPERTS AND LISTENING:

Chances are that you are not an expert in your new endeavor, and you will need to put yourself on a steep learning curve. This, of course, is what makes it so scintillating and fun. Advisors, coaches, experts, use them. Build up an arsenal of people with a lot of know-how, and don't be afraid to pick their brains. There is no honor is repeating mistakes that already have great solutions. Use the known solutions and move on to failing at the tough stuff.

PROCESS FOR DAMAGE CONTROL:

The fit will hit the shan.

That's life. You will spend some of your years on this planet rebuilding things. I have met too many people along this life journey who have become defined by their tragic events. Their story almost always begins with "I used to be..." Mentally, it's important to understand that the things that you have and hold dear all have a life-span. They die, they go out of fashion, they get replaced by better technology. Markets crash, economies fail, legislation changes. Accidents happen. The best in the world are prepared for this. They have the right insurance, they also have the ability to roll up the sleeves and get back to building. Being process driven, they enjoy the process and can derive pleasure from their restarts. Since the only constant is change, it's imperative that you fortify your mind to accept loss, and to accept changes in prestige and status.

PROCESS FOR KEEPING YOUR EGO IN CHECK:

Humility, especially early in your career, is what allows you to fail, and fail the right way. If you can get yourself to the point where you are willing to fail as many times as it takes to get to where you can master the idea, then you will be well on your way to actually getting it done.

PROCESS FOR MANAGING YOUR RESOURCES:

It's hard to be brilliant when you are broke. I am not saying there is anything wrong with working two jobs and grinding like a beast to get by, but realistically, this should be temporary as you build and establish yourself. Remember also that you HAVE to make time to be building your skill set, and that this is a priority item. Your number one resource is you, and if it is being run around bussing tables all week, it's hard to imagine you getting that high-utility skill set down. So, manage your time, your cash and your growth. And do it well.

PROCESS FOR ENTERING THE DRAGON'S LAIR:

That's right. Since we are building up a version of you that is going to go out and give a few dragons a pretty bad day, it makes sense to make sure we have a good process for getting up the courage to go in and deal with our fears.

It definitely helps to remind yourself that this has already been conquered by someone, and therefore it most certainly is possible. Getting up the courage to make the tough calls, to grab destiny by the balls and forge ahead to build your vision is as critical a skill as any mentioned thus far. A good idea without the steel to follow through vanishes like a puff of smoke in a high winds storm. Have a method of going to greet your biggest fears head on.

PROCESS FOR BEING OPPORTUNISTIC

They literally are everywhere, opportunities. Particularly in your head. People with great attitudes are always finding new adventures and new ways to create with new groups of people. People with a bad mindset spend a whole lot of time thinking about what they don't have, what they could have had and being bored and unhappy. That is a choice. I have seen people pull themselves literally out of the gutter, and it's beyond a proven fact that it can be done, provided you are actively pulling.

PROCESS FOR CREATING AND MANAGING ENERGY

Energy. Its big business. Red bull. Five-hour energy. Chevron. Tesla. Starbucks. They all have one thing in common. They sell energy. It's what the world relies on.

You have a finite amount of it. Approximately 80 years' worth. How you spend it is going to be a critical metric in your life. You most definitely want to become an expert at producing, storing, and managing it. This includes when you sleep, what you drink, what you do to rest and recover, and how big you let yourself dream. How easily do you get distracted, and end up spending time on other things? How much energy can you spend in the pain zone?

At its most basic, life is 100% about managing energy. What you eat affects your energy. What you feel like you should spend your time on consumes energy. What thoughts you linger on, and choose to spend time on, this also is a choice on how to spend energy. The people you hang out with, they also consume your energetic resources. The simplest equation is that however much energy you spend towards your goal, generally equates to how much you get out of it.

Being motivated can be described as a higher energy state. You can do more in these higher energy states. Frustration too is a higher energy state and can also lead to breakthrough thinking. Decisions, and determined action are forms of higher energy and lead to measurable outcomes. All in all, you need to be in control of this process, and you need to be extremely good at choosing how you spend your energy. It is a finite resource, and anyone who does anything awesome will need to display PhD level expertise.

PROCESS FOR "THE BURN"

Almost everyone I have ever met cares about outcomes. People become upset and destabilized when things don't go their way. This makes sense, as the saying goes: "Show me someone who is good at losing and I'll show you a loser." People get agitated, they have tantrums, and they behave as if someone has set their soul on fire.

I like to call this moment the BURN. Here is the thing. There are a lot of moments in life that can lead to the BURN, but the real question is "how long should it last?"

One of the biggest lessons to learn in life is that many things are not going to go your way, but by being a consistently PROCESS DRIVEN person, and staying the course, you are going to get results. You are going to have to become a 12th Degree Dan Grandmaster at dealing with these unexpected and variant outcomes. YES. You will be aggravated. And Burning.

You have to develop a method that allows you to analyze what went wrong, look for solutions, do damage control, and then set new coordinates, establish emotional closure and move on. Period. Developing this practice is a wonderful way of taking control of your emotions after difficult events. We know that certain events will take longer than others, losing a loved one is not something you can set an alarm clock for 1 hour from now and then write some notes and get on with it. Someone rejecting you for prom is. This should not lead to locking yourself in a room for a week, dying all your clothes black and writing songs about spiders.

Once you understand that failures, setbacks and stubborn obstacles are part of the problem, it's quite easy to understand that you will be required to work through them, and you will need your own ingenuity, your own changes and modifications in order to have a better attempt at the next one.

PROCESS FOR UNDERSTANDING WHAT IS LIKELY TO BREAK DOWN

Each reader of this book has different emotional make ups. We all break down at different spots along the journey. Understanding what is likely to break down and when allows you to build some contingencies, have some experts on standby or avoid known treacherous territory. Some of the most successful people I know are the most volatile and have the most personality glitches. But what has made them great is that they have found answers to their breakdowns and have developed techniques to minimize negative outcomes.

PROCESS FOR UNDERSTANDING WAVE CYCLES IN LIFE:

Nothing happens in a linear fashion. Generally, things work in waves. Waves have some important technical aspects which we will repurpose for our own understanding of human performance.

Crests: Top of the wave, best performance, highlights, top achievement.

Trough: Rock bottom, worst feeling ever, things not even close to going according to plan.

Amplitude: Height of your crest or trough from your median line. When the guy who is ranked 500 in the world suddenly wins a grand slam, this crest has a huge amplitude-it's miles away from his median line.

Wavelength: Distance between each crest and trough.

Median line: This is your general line. This is where you spend the vast majority of your time. This is the average between your great highs and your super lows.

Let's put this into a visual example. Let's take Sally who is trying to build herself into someone who works out more.

1. Get all geared up and motivated and get going: Buy special containers to cook all your food, join gym, buy special neoprene gym gear, etc.

2. Have a great first month, start feeling some change come over your body, lose a few pounds, ask your friends if they see a difference.

3. Give yourself a couple of days off because of kids homework assignments, accept invitation to join the guys or ladies for a few drinks. Skip some workouts. Have sudden work deadline, stress causes you to overeat.

4. Suddenly you have not been working out for 6 weeks, longer than you worked out for.

5. Push feelings of guilt to back of mind, gain confidence from sentences like, "I know I can do this, it's just the timing is not right."

6. Wake up and feel really bad that you "have no mental toughness and discipline."

Let's Plot her progress in a simple diagram.

JANUARY	FEBRUARY	MARCH	APRIL	MAY	JUNE
X X	X	X X	X	X	
X X X	X	X X		X X	
X	X X	X	X	X	X X X
X X X	X	X X X X			

If you look at it through the lens of a longer time scale, as well as the idea that this is something that will most likely happen in waves, not in a perfect linear form, then you can look at the whole and take some data, but also psychologically allow yourself to course correct.

For some of us we have a built in mentality that if it's not perfect, then we don't want it at all, and so when we look at April here, a month where we only worked out 2 times- for most of us we would be so disappointed in ourselves, that this is where most of us would give up.

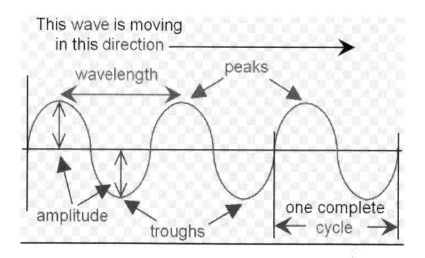

Looking at life, learning, self-improvement as a wave function, and we look back at our workout log, we start to see things emerging a little differently. We start to see that what we did a good job of in our 6-month log is to keep the DIRECTION of the wave in place. We were moving forward nicely. We see that we had more amplitude in some months, meaning we worked out more, and had a high positive amplitude which means we are moving our wave forward.

Wavelength is the amount of time we keep the good workout routine, and we see some waves were longer than others which is completely normal and acceptable.

We see the distance between the troughs and the amplitude of the toughs. This is what you have to watch out for - 6 weeks of eating pizza only and feeling sorry for yourself, whilst drinking beers and donuts only would result in a very long trough, with a super high amplitude. Not good!!!!

Right now, our first candidate should be feeling pretty good about themselves, and rather than quitting, they should be looking to course correct just slightly.

Imagine their total of 32 workouts over a six-month period. With course correcting, they aim to add one per month in the next 6-month period--

That brings them up to 38 workouts in the next wave. Instead of quitting, they have had a pretty good year. We take a deep look into the motivational factors here, because they have not done enough to move the needle in the direction of looking like a cover model on a magazine. And this realization can often get people to ask "Well, why put all this effort in?"

Again, the answers should not be made by the ego.

PERCEPTION: If I don't end up with a six pack, then it's not worth it.

REALITY: 180 pound you is healthier than 200 pound you. Because you feel good after a workout. Because you are getting all the benefits that exercise has for you. Because you are conditioning your brain to build lifelong habits.

There is no accident in success. You read stories about how much money entrepreneurs and big companies spend on getting their product right, how much money they spend interviewing, watching people do the thing they are trying to make a product for, designing advertising campaigns, etc. If you want to be successful, you will absolutely have to follow the following guidelines:

1. You need to help humanity: There are very few products that won't be consumed by humans. Even products for animals will be bought by a human, and that human needs to be willing to buy your product. What are you giving them? Happiness, a tool? A moment of relief? Figure out what it is that you are giving them.

2. Be willing to work hard.

3. Be willing to be consistent.

4. Be willing to adapt.

5. Be willing to recruit help: You cannot do it alone, and therefore you will want other passionate people to help you build your dream.

6. Be a humanist, if you love the idea that someone using your product is going to feel amazing, and their day just got a little better, then you will be inspired to bring that product into their lives!

7. Be good at developing partnerships: It is incredible the power of other people's ideas. You will definitely benefit from having other people's creative energy help toward your projects.

8. Be a long-term thinker and planner. Think out, about 100 years from now: hopefully your design will not kill the planet. Point yourself in a direction that facilitates a growing relationship with the world, and a growing application of wisdom. These are critically important if we hope to align ourselves with the idea of an even better world in 100 years!

There are a vast number of personalities and stemming from these traits are a vast number of different methods to get things done. With practice and refinement, you will slowly nail down a method that is right for you and begin to master the art of building a reliable, result yielding process. No matter how good your ideas or your plan, it remains largely due to your processes that you keep moving forward and consistently taking the actions that lead to sustainable results.

Chapter 6: The Roadblocks

Every year, billions of people set their goals and aspirations for the upcoming year. Sadly, a huge number of these goals will never be achieved. Wouldn't it be fun to meet with a top actuary from one of the bigger insurance companies and ask him to come up with the actual percentage of goals set, versus goals achieved. You should be well aware at the outset that the odds are against you actually reaching the goal, extinction is the rule and survival is the exception. This makes beating the system all the more enjoyable!

With the best of intentions, most of us start the journey towards achievement positive and hyped up, raring to go. Somewhere, out there, lurking in the shadows is a potential pitfall, a potential item that can derail you, set you on the path to failure, or stop you dead in your tracks. Some of these are external and uncontrollable, but the vast majority are internal and controllable. We cannot predict when we will be confronted by some of the bigger external roadblocks. We will also be challenged to work hard and make as much progress as possible in dealing effectively with our internal roadblocks.

This Chapter is about trying to identify some of the more common road-blocks. It is important to understand the following concepts and their effect on drive and motivation and to be fully prepared for how to deal with them. We want to deliver answers that can be deeply embedded in our PROCESS for how to deal with certain roadblocks and keep moving forward.

1. Poor Decision Making

The events of our lives don't control our lives. Decisions do.

There are two elements that go into decision making. The first one is having the knowledge and education base. You cannot make educated decisions if you don't have the know-how. The second element is being able to apply that knowledge. Even if you do have the knowledge, does your emotional make up allow you to take the action of applying it.

Brain Chemistry plays a big role when people make poor decisions in emotionally charged situations. When we become excited or fearful, our prefrontal cortex, which is used for logical thinking shuts down. The amygdala, the primal, animal part of the brain takes over. Your frame of reference can go completely out of whack, and you enter the immediate survival, it's-you-or-me mode, rather than strategizing over long-term wellbeing.

Fight or flight instinct can be extremely useful, as in situations where you actually need to survive, but it can be extremely debilitating if you are triggered to be in fight-or-flight mode, but it's actually just a regular, everyday situation. Simply put, if a cobra jumps out at you and you reach for an ashtray to throw at it, it makes sense. If are tempted to throw a football at your TV because the Steelers just missed a catch right in the end zone, chances are, amygdala is kicking in.

From a chemistry point of view, that heightened state of panic does not last long, and if you give the amygdala a chance to calm down, the prefrontal cortex can kick in again and your decision making will drastically improve.

For most of us, here is the golden rule: try not to make any life changing moves in these heightened emotional situations. Put up some barriers to decision making and try to delay making any decisions until a later time. For athletes, make sure your routines kick in, and you work through rehearsed decisions, and 10 000 repetition strong scenarios, relying on the myelin sheath coating and not the amygdala.

2. The allure of success.

When you have built good habits and you are starting to roll, you start to make escalations. What was once 10 pushups is now 1 hour of chest workouts, 4 times a week interspersed with superb nutrition, and all your other training blocks: legs, back, shoulders, endurance etc.

Your days are hard. You wake up and you have big items to check off the to do list. You are busy. It's tough. It's a grind.

You start to see some big success, you now have the mansion, the Lambos, the iced-up Rolex. You built the greatest pool ever seen, with a seemingly endless pool party that is still continuing. Suddenly you day has changed. What used to be getting up at 5 to go and workout has become going to bed at 5.

Success can have a profound impact on your day and can kick out the habits and routines that got you there in the first place. Many a great achiever has been seduced by the smooth gleaming allure of success.

For most people to stay a success, they still need to continue the hard-daily grind.

The amount of sheer work that it takes for a top athlete or businessman/businesswoman to stay at the top of the game is not only mind boggling, it's also continuous. In order to stay a number 1, you have to continue to behave like a number 1, and you cannot suddenly start spending all your days on the golf course. Working at that level takes enormous planning and execution. The top performers have very little time to enjoy the fruits of their labor.

For anyone who is genuinely interested in success, and genuinely interested in creating something that has meaning, your lifestyle is going to consist of hard days, and hard years. Your only real reward will be the daily sense of accomplishment.

3. The seemingly never-ending daily grind.

Just as success can derail your daily grind, the hard work itself can become a road-block. There is an unknown quantity in there. How long will it actually take to reach this goal? 5 years? 10 years? 20? Having a set timeframe, like when you start a college degree helps. Med school is going to be 8-11 years approx. This makes it at least a little easier to metabolize internally. Entrepreneurs, athletes who might work for years and years before the pay-off, need to have vast pools of motivation and belief in order to make themselves do the work consistently as the years tick on.

Generally, we are reluctant to have the discomfort of a day that is tough from start to finish. We will tolerate this for a certain time, but as time rolls by, we inevitably will question our method, our talents, abilities and resolve.

I think there is no better story than Nelson Mandela, the great South African leader who spent 27 years in jail before finally being released to lead the country. He was offered a return to his family many times, a chance to have all charges dismissed, a chance to see his wife and daughters. It must have been excruciating to see his family move on, graduate, get married and not be a part of those experiences. And I am sure he had days where he was oh-so-close- to quitting and just signing the necessary documents. How difficult would the thought be of spending all that time in prison and missing essentially his whole life if eventually his effort was for nothing? That one thought alone would have made many people decide that the fight was not for them, and that the risks were just too extreme. He was fighting for an enormous cause, he found his motivation in the possibility to positively impact millions of oppressed South Africans, and he stayed the hard road. 27 years of it. Finally, he reached his goal and vision, and the walls of Apartheid came crashing down to the thunderous will of one man, powered by the need for self-expression and freedom of millions. And perhaps there is no finer example of the raw power of human will to create powerful, positive change.

Most of us do not have enough passion for what we are doing to make it worthwhile, and most of us do not have enough belief that we will bring our vision to reality.

For most of us, that horrifying moment where we give up on our dreams and settle for the more convenient life, the easy way and the creature comforts of the known road is so subtle, it's like a feather glancing across a Mack Truck, but that whispery soft touch is enough to permanently send the truck down a different road.

4. Scattering.

Success does not happen in a linear measurable way- one success after another, making it easy to measure progress. Sometimes doing the right thing actually takes us backwards before we go forward, and sometimes the little victories are there, but they are interspersed with plenty of failure. You can see that the idea has merit, but plenty of work still needs to be done to make the idea into a consistent, result-wielding powerhouse. You need to have excellent staying power to work through these parts of your career where there are no immediate gains, and you have to balance the idea of trusting your process and just slogging it out or realizing this is the time to make some changes and adapt your process to trigger something new to happen. This non-linear process can derail a lot of people. Take being an entrepreneur for example. Most of the really successful ones that I know have gone bust more than once already. And for most people, this would be intolerable. Your only sure-fire way to deal with this is through rugged building of your confidence and knowledge base. If you feel like you are getting good at your trade, while you have a lot of confidence and trust in your work ethic, your character traits, then you can nurture belief. Belief, and hanging onto your vision can make all the difference at the end of the day. Your final arrow in the quiver is passion. If there is a part of you that would do what you are doing anyway, even if you didn't get paid eventually, that secretly enjoys the challenge, and enjoys the grind

5. Shade.

Not everyone is as excited about your new habits and success as you are, and for reasons such as jealousy, or feeling bad that they are falling behind you, there can be negative feedback from certain members of your family, peer group, work environment. I have actually seen it where someone really steps up their game and ends up being fired because of it. The reason: their boss feels that if left for too long, the new habits will be noticed by top brass, and could lead to them being judged negatively. They don't want a new prize stallion in their office, they want someone good, but not as good as them.

Pretty much all the way until you actually do something, you will have people telling you it can't be done, and that you are insane for trying, and that the journey is just too hard.

6. Linking

We have all dealt with setbacks and negative experiences in our lives.

They all have their own impact on our perceptions, and each one registers a certain amount of pain and discomfort in your memory. Someone who has had a real or perceptually negative experience with something, will have a harder time getting motivated for something than someone who had the same experience, but remembers or processed it less painfully.

What happens with linking, is that you re-experience a number of feelings at the same time. Imagine thinking of your worst sport loss, a death in the family, your worst break up, your most embarrassing moment, all at the same time. With linking, this is exactly what happens. Those experiences are linked together, and when one feeling is triggered, it automatically triggers emotions related to those other experiences. We can often see this as an overly emotional response to something relatively mundane.

Let's see how this works a little bit more. Imaginary feelings can be just as powerful as real experiences. Someone who is in love with a tv character, feels every bit as in love as someone who is in love with a real person. How you perceive the world is largely an imaginary state. Someone who feels like things always go wrong, might have some factual reasons behind how this feeling developed, (in reality things do not always go wrong, they also go right very often) but this feeling is what shapes the reality of the person holding it. It is not uncommon for someone with a negative bias to greet the day, feeling that they are destined to experience something negative, and life therefore becomes something they are fearful of.

Remember it's not important how real it is, but rather the individual's perception of it-

1. Let's say that bob moves tries to start his own business. He works 18 hours a day for a year and this is a 7/10 powerful negative experience for him.

2. He invests his life savings. Having to deal with having no disposable income and the stress of potentially losing his savings is a negative experience for him.

3. Finally, the business starts failing and he has to go through the legal red-tape of shutting it down and filing bankruptcy.

4. He also needs to find a job, so he starts interviewing and the thought of having to work for 3 years for someone else again while rebuilding his savings is a particularly intense negative feeling.

Now imagine Bob lost a girlfriend because of his entrepreneurial spirit and had been told by someone very meaningful to him that his life choices and trying to follow his dreams is reckless, irresponsible and downright silly.

Whenever poor Bob thinks about following a dream again, it links him to all of these negative feelings. Chasing a dream to Bob means the following: loss of savings, friends turning on you, girlfriends heading for the exit, legal nightmares.

Imagine for a minute how motivated Bob will be when he thinks of his next entrepreneurial idea. It might come as no surprise when he has little to zero ability to get himself to take the risk again.

Let's Science this bad bot a little bit: Inside your brain, you have a process where pathways that carry neurological signals become more and more grooved. Imagine a river delta. There are many pathways that the water can flow over. But the thickest one is going to carry the most water. It's more easily accessible.

When this happens inside your brain, you end up with neural pathways that are more easily accessible than others. When you think certain thoughts over and over again, it becomes easier and easier to think these thoughts, as your brain builds a habit of thinking them, and you we get what's called a "coating of the myelin sheath"

Medical Definition of myelin sheath: the insulating covering that surrounds an axon with multiple spiral layers of myelin, that is discontinuous at the nodes of Ranvier, and that increases the speed at which a nerve impulse can travel along an axon — called also *medullary sheath*

This super highway that the nerve impulse can travel along is a wonderful asset when it comes to triggering habits related

131

to performance of your skill set, but it can be a problem when each road is connected to a deep pool of negative emotion.

Now, whenever you have a negative experience, you are feeling multiple past negative experiences at the same time. We can often see this expressed as massive over-reaction to something. "You get super upset over the little things" would be a common expression you have probably heard if you are one of these folks.

Positive linking: We all have this linking process in some form or another. There are certain people who are able to be intensely resilient under almost any condition. This is because just about every situation you throw at them links to their resilient feeling. They may even seek out difficult situations, because they enjoy this resilient feeling so much, and they want avenues to express it.

There are many examples of this, and we could most likely find an example of each emotion and someone who has an overabundance of it.

Linking can have immediate and long-term results on your confidence and performance. We can see athletes who have a strong of close losses, suddenly start to break down in decision making, and start to lose confidence. This is directly related to an increase in fear of a negative result, as the immediate history tells them that the outcome in this situation has been predominantly negative and that if their 2-10 past performance continues, then they should expect another failure here. This perception creates an altered emotional environment, and often triggers a self-fulfilling prophecy of yet another loss.

The dieter actually creates a negative emotional environment internally as they link to past failures, and their previous attempts and failures at dieting, and with each day that unfolds, the pressure internally increases and the fear that they will regress or fail increases until it is actually easier internally to simply fail than it is to continue to forge ahead with their nutrition plan.

7. How you respond to pressure

Once you have done the really hard work of practicing something a million times, it then becomes about building and developing composure and the ability to perform the action regardless of the situation. In other words, it's about forgetting the occasion.

It is important to be able to reflect on how you think and perform under pressure- and by this same measure, it's important to be able to recognize what skills you need to work on to become better at handling these situations. You would be amazed at how few people have any type of plan for how to improve in these areas, and end up addressing pressure in the same way, again and again.

The general blueprint for responding to pressure.

- First thing is to **ASSESS** the situation. What type of crisis are you having?

- Next you will want to **TAKE STOCK** of your resources. What are the things you have that you can put to work? Things like your breathing, your body language, your decisions, your affirmations. The things you can control, it is imperative that you begin to bring them inline and online.

- You now need to make a **PLAN** of how to use your resources to alter the situations as you had previously assessed it.

- A key element here is knowing what will make the situation worse. Not all action actually leads to solutions. Your analysis should definitely include actions to stay away from. Finally, **EXECUTE** your decisions.

8. Loss of momentum

- There is no more powerful motivator than progress. You will feel better about just about anything if you have some momentum. If you are on a track, and moving along it, and you have some results, and a system of habits that supports even more momentum.

- Unfortunately, sometimes we plateau. Sometimes we make mistakes. Sometimes life throws us a curve ball. Things that were not caused by us, have a dramatic effect on us. The decisions we make in response to these unforseens, surprises and obstacles is what will ultimately create our outcomes. I will always remember my coach saying, **"The problem is not your problem. Your response to the problem is your problem."**

- One of the crucial things to understand about life is the dance between cause and effect. You have the chance to be the "cause" of an "effect", but simultaneously life has the ability to "cause" "effects" on you. You are in control of a lot of decisions, a lot of choices, but you also have no control over certain outcomes, and you need to be able to navigate your way to success with this being the "field" that you navigate your way through.

- Loss of momentum through plateauing, through unforeseen events and surprises has been the ultimate roadblock for all too many people. They get stuck in a wrong channel of thinking, they become negative, the road between expectation and reality starts to widen, and their system becomes destabilized. What's needed is to create a new paradigm by jolting the system out of the "current known" and create new feelings through renewed ideas, planning and information.

9. Procrastination

We have all heard the sentence- "You can do it!" a million times. And for the most part it's true= we can just about achieve anything we set our minds to. How close or how far away from this achievement we are is a matter for another debate. (Many a person has turned back thinking they will never get there when in actual fact they are quite close!)

One of the key differentiating factors in achievement is whether or not you "BELIEVE" you can achieve the thing you are after. One of the greatest causative factors in Procrastination is this point. Let's be fair here- IF you absolutely believed that by starting this diet, and getting in great shape, you will not only succeed, but also be approached by a modeling agency and be offered a million-dollar contract within the next six months- wouldn't you be ultra-motivated to do it? I would be off the couch right away.

What if you just looked at the number of people who are in great shape, and said that the body is just physics- and if you provide the right chemistry (or lack of it- think- hold back on the chocolates!!!) your body will respond by changing shape just as it has done for millions of people. Ok- simple enough. Then why aren't you in great shape?

What leads you to doubt that the physics will work for you. What leads you to doubt that you can be consistent and finish the course?

What makes you eat the cheap calorie and break the healthy cycle? What makes you overindulge?

At the heart of failure lie two distinct root causes.

1. Belief- If you don't believe you will succeed, you will be far more vulnerable to the opportunities to break course or succumb to temptation.

2. Procrastination-- Many a diet is starting in a few days' time, or next week, or soon- many a great habit is just around the corner from being well formed. Many a great achievement is in the head waiting to come out!

I was lucky enough to catch an AA meeting and to find out the most common problem with addiction is the idea that the drug addict has that they can stop anytime they want to. They are in control of their habit.

I noticed the correlation between this, and the person addicted to mediocrity. The only difference is the addiction.

Addicted to your safe current situation? Not really desperate to get going? Thinking what difference could a week or two make? What's one more chocolate going to do? Staying up an hour extra won't really hurt that bad?

Your new diet, workout plan, business venture, studying something new, looking for opportunity- it does not matter- if you have succumbed to any of those thoughts or actions- then you have probably procrastinated!

SO- with that being said, let's get back to the opening sentence for this chapter- You can do it. Fact.

You should do it.

It's going to feel absolutely incredibly amazing if you do it!

So- Let's get out there and get it going!

10. Emotional betrayal. The biggest brute of them all, Fear.

Betrayal. It has been the cornerstone of some of the most famous movies, books, pieces of literature. Stories throughout history. It has probably happened to everyone reading this book at least once- somewhere. "Et-Tu Brute? – You bloody bastard!!"

Of course, as you might have guessed by now- we are going to turn the magnifying glass inward and ask the simple question-- are you betraying yourself! Are you the Brutus to your Caesar?

If you give up on your dreams- what's left?

The threat of success. We have all heard of self-sabotage and we have all probably had the same thought- which is-- "why? Why would success be the one thing that people are afraid of. Why would they take actions to stop themselves from achieving the very success they are looking for? What a horrible affliction to have- snatching defeat from the jaws of victory- stopping yourself from achieving things that matter to you because at some deep psychological level you won't let yourself have them.   And yet this is far more common than most people know, far more common than most people like to believe.

You will succumb to the greater fear.

Fear is going to be one of the more important characters in our life and in our society. We have to be extremely thoughtful if we are to develop an understanding of how and why fear is dictating our decisions.

Further into this discussion, we will address how people who understand our fears are able to manipulate them against us, or use them to cause us to take action, normally to buy a product.

"People can be afraid of just about anything: afraid of truth, afraid of fortune, afraid of each other" Remarked the late great Ralph Waldo Emerson.

I would go so far as to add to this list: people are afraid of risk, of commitment, of hard work, of change, of being brave, of loving fully, of failure. They have a deep fear of rejection.

In reality Fear is something that we can actually be taught. Growing up in Racist, Apartheid era south Africa, this was most definitely the order of the day. All the propaganda, instruction from teachers in schools and general atmosphere created was- "you should fear the black man- he is dangerous"

Fear, for the most part is a learned behavior. If I was to take an unguided walk through a dense patch of amazon jungle, I would be surrounded by dangers I did not even know existed. The killer wasps, piranhas, crocodiles, stinging plants and strange bacteria. All just waiting for the chance to find some open wound, a change to turn me into a delicious tasty lunch. I would be incredibly hesitant to go in there. I would have a very real fear of death, underpinned by the fact that I have no idea what dangerous species is lurking ready to kill me, and the fact that if I do encounter any of these little fellas, I would have no idea how to deal with them.

You can easily imagine me walking through the forest with my tail between my legs, shaking uncontrollably and muttering under my breath "this is the dumbest idea ever, who in their right minds would want to do this? I must have meatballs for brains if this is how I get to spend my day!"

Now let's contrast this with Steve Irwin, the crocodile hunter.

A cobra pops its head up. He looks calmly at it "Ooohhh, she is a beauty, she's looking right at me. Good on ya mate." He grabs it by the neck and gives it a little kiss on the head, before putting it back in the wild, and going on to catch a crocodile.

The vastly different interpretation and subsequent action in these two scenarios is mostly because of education. Steve has been playing with crocodiles and cobras for a while. He understands them and has learned their behaviors and what to watch out for. This makes him much less susceptible to fear.

KNOWLEDGE is a great antidote to fear.

Fear can be a great antidote to progress. It can seep into our mind like a poison, robbing us of ambition, sleep, good relationships. It can also be contagious.

In trying to understand fear, a famous experiment done on monkeys (Susan Mineka 1985) showed that lab reared monkeys did not fear snakes, while monkeys raised in the wild did. What was interesting here is that not all monkeys could have had a bad experience with a snake, and so we would have expected some deviation in behavior, but the fear of snakes was completely pervasive in the wild.

Contrasted to the lab reared monkeys, ruled out the idea that there was a genetic predisposition, as they had no fear at all.

What then happened is even more interesting, the lab monkeys when put with the nature-reared monkeys, learned by watching that the nature monkeys did not reach for food when a snake was near, and so became conditioned to fear snakes.

When they were brought back into the lab, and tested three months later, this fear persisted, indicating that not only are a response to our past traumas, but also to fears we learn from parents and friends.

Yes, that's right! You could be living someone else's fear! Fear that is not even your own- think about how silly that is for a second. Because someone else has inhibitions, and they are super afraid, they have gone on and passed those on to you, and you are now super reactive to them! Does that not sound like the most asinine thing in the world?

The road to success is going to have many roadblocks, and there will be challenges that you could not imagine or could not possible have been prepared for. There will be outside causes that derail you, set you back, push you completely off course. You will have varying amounts of willpower, inner strength and brilliant decision making. But the one thing you have to do, is endure. Change is constant, and not even the most ardent roadblock can last forever. Not even the most daunting, damaging, destructive events will last forever. There is always a workaround, a fix, a solution and a way to move forward and past.

CHAPTER 7: MOTIVATION

Motivation. Stoked. Lit. Rocking and rolling.

Wouldn't it be nice if every time you were feeling lazy, you could flip a switch and enter a ultra-high energy state? Something that would cause goosebumps that could give your arm hairs a perm. A shiver runs down the spine, you pop the collar and head straight out the door. You'd get the same look from your friends as the caveman who first discovered fire (I suggest taking this out).

Motivation is a huge and complex subject, and involves every human feeling, both intrinsic and extrinsic. Why do we idolize sports stars so much? Why are we starstruck by people who climb Everest? Why are we fascinated by serial killers? Strange crimes? The answer to all of these is that it's hard to wrap your head around the motivation required to perform some of these extreme acts. It's hard to perfectly account for the balance of impulse, sheer will and environmental factors that can either make you act or resist taking it.

(Take out): Who in their right minds wants to be freezing like a popsicle at 30,000 feet in gale force winds in one of those mini tents, held together by flexi-rods? What drives some athletes to be at the top of their games for nearly 20 years? Why were they not tempted to say, "no more jets, no more 6-hour training days, no more weird menus? I am just going to stop now and enjoy my success, enjoy my 25,000 square foot home. It's time to relax now!"

(Take out): Finally, how do some of the world's most prolific criminals cross over the threshold and actually act on their idea? Imagine yourself dressed in a cat-burglar nylon suit, hot and sweaty, a nervous wreck, deep wedgie, about to scale a 20-foot building and dance your way through the field of lasers, to make a grab at the Cullinan Diamond. It feels like ants are crawling on your neck, carotid artery pulsing. You are scratching, sweating, hyperventilating. Finally, you quit: "No, bollocks to this idea, I am going home."

We all instinctively appreciate the amount of motivation necessary to take certain actions. We can understand the extraordinary lengths the human emotional system can stretch to. We have ample evidence that with the right motivation, very close to anything is possible. Building a billion-dollar business, someone has done it. Win 20 grand slams, someone has done it. Scale highest mountain, tick here please, done and dusted.

Knowing that the most massive goals imaginable are achievable, and that someone has probably already achieved them, should be very good news for us. We know that if we can understand and nurture our motivation, we really can achieve that dream that's been rolling around our heads. Sadly, most of our motivation is used to do what we NEED to do: work, pay the bills, and maintain our lifestyle. But it can be hard to find the motivation to go the extra mile and do the things our dreams require us to do.

Understanding how motivation works is the crucible to success. Understanding how we build it, trigger it, how we lose it. Understanding and mastery of your own motivational system will no doubt have a dramatic impact on your life. So, what exactly is motivation? Is it a thought? A Feeling? A State of being? Imagine a seesaw with a marble on it. Right now, it's completely tilted to one side, the marble is totally stationary at the bottom in the corner. You are in an idle state, sitting in your chair at home. Suddenly, you start to get a little pang of hunger. The see-saw vibrates and the little marble wobbles ever so slightly. You wait 20 mins. Now that little pang of hunger has gotten much stronger. Suddenly the seesaw starts to move, and the marble starts rolling in the other direction. As soon as that marble is on its way to the other side, it starts to feel easier to get up than it did to stay put on the couch just moments earlier. You get up off the couch and go make a sandwich.

Each and every choice that we make comes with a price-tag. In other words, at some point, it is easier to change than to stay the same. Somehow, we cross a mental threshold and the see saw begins to swing to the other side. And now it feels more compelling and easier to actually do the work, than to sit with the self-loathing and disappointment of not doing it.

(Take out) It is easier to act and feel lonely than it is to stay with the abusive boyfriend. It is easier to feel awkward while interviewing for a new job than to feel disappointed about your dwindling bank account.

So, let's take a more complex example. We will use Bob and his twin brother Errol. Bob has two fears, the fear of rejection and the fear of loneliness. Because he has a deeper fear of rejection, he cannot bear the idea of asking someone out, even if it means that he will be activating his other fear of loneliness.

We flip the script and Bob's twin brother Errol has the same fears but is far more afraid of loneliness than rejection. He has the same two fears, just in different quantities. He is able to overcome his fear of rejection and go speak to some potential dates as well as make some friends, as the deeper fear of loneliness is what's driving his actions.

You may think, well, what a lucky boy Errol is, that he has those 2 fears in their different quantities the way he has. His way allows him to move forward while his poor brother is held captive. Bobs marble rolls towards not taking action, and Errol's marble rolls towards action.

Perhaps there is a little bit of luck insofar as the setting the stage is concerned. But the real homework comes in being able to move the marble to where you need it, when you need it.

We all know there are many things that can move your marble,

Fear can make it move,

Greed can make it move,

Sensing an opportunity can make it move,

Love and passion can make it move.

Routine and discipline can make it move.

Acting on good or bad information can make it move.

Desperation can make it move.

Psychologists describe this as: the set of psychological factors that need to be present in order for someone to act. We can go one step further and describe that as a need that requires satisfaction. Those needs of course can also be wants, and those needs or wants can be acquired through society, circle of friends, rewards, or simple lifestyle. So, then the real question becomes: What moves your marble? Know the answer to this, and suddenly the world of your goals and dreams becomes a much different place.

With control of your motivators, you dictate where the marble rolls. You can get the marble to roll enough to get you in the gym, to put the time into being a good parent, a good husband, a good mother, to resist overspending, to put down the chocolate, to search for resolutions instead of just throwing in the towel, to go work for NASA. You decide your own destiny. We can create feelings with our thinking, and we can create motivation with our thinking. In other words, the most motivated people are closer to the one or two thoughts that motivate them than other people. They know their 'why'.

THE INNER WORKINGS OF MOTIVATION

Ok. Let's dig in. Let's take a look at some of the building blocks of great motivation. We would be well rewarded if we could find the common threads in the actions of persons that have tremendous motivation. We don't need to re-invent the world of motivation just to be able to copy those who have already achieved great mastery over it. We want the house of your dreams to be built not on foundations of sand, but instead the solid granite that is: work ethic held in place by great motivation.

THE PROCESS OF MOTIVATION

The start:

1. **Friction and inertia:** The biggest common fallacy surrounding motivation is that you need to somehow build it up before you start something. The hard part, the high friction element, is in the beginning, getting started. Once you overcome that particular hurdle, it gets a lot easier. What successful people often

instinctively put to use is the idea of automating the start of an action. They leave themselves no outs, no dialogue, no escape routes. When the alarm goes off they start. What they do is they AUTOMATE the start and they use routines to do it. This way they are able to overcome inertia. IF you arrive at the start of an action believing you still have a choice, then it will be easy to make the alternative choice of working out tomorrow or starting later in the day. We definitely do not want this. We want it to be a: "It's happening right now, no if's, but's or maybe's!" We need to tap into some discipline and some habit building to schedule the new behavior. Writing, gym, starting a business are all going to need you to build a set time that you stick to early on. Without this, you will leave the start point as an unknown, and will probably not get around to it. You MUST set aside a time for the new behavior and groove this time into a habit. I.E, you always go to gym right after work. This brings us to our second important piece: You cannot rely on willpower, you need to rely on planning, scheduling and habit building skills. Setting a schedule is the best way to give birth to new behaviors. It creates the time and environment in which they will live. Lastly, trying to decide where or when to work is a fool's errand. You will spend the vast majority of your time trying to solve that riddle and probably never actually get around to just simply doing the work. Set a schedule. Take the daily decision making out of the equation. Have it on your scheduler, and when that alarm goes off, literally just stand up and start doing it. Once this beast has been put onto automation, there is a far greater chance of you actually following through, even when your motivation levels are low. Professionals set a schedule and stick to it, and amateurs wait for motivation and inspiration to come floating magically to them in the air.

2. **Motivation generally comes AFTER we begin a behavior, not BEFORE**. Another secret of the master of motivation is that they know they will actually only start feeling good and getting the flood of motivation, AFTER they arrive at the gym, and are working through their warm-up. Many of my best ever training sessions would never have happened, had it not been for routine and ritual. The number of mornings you wake up at 5am and say "I don't want to do this" is probably 50%. You do it anyway, and then suddenly 45 minutes into your workout, you find a high gear and produce some of your best work. It would be a crime to have listened to that early voice and just stayed in bed. And for most people, they are so much closer to success than they think: conquering inertia and understanding that motivation is probably not going to be the thing that gets you out of bed are key elements to getting going.

3. **The power of Ritual.** Waking up, pulling on your socks, packing your gym bag, picking your favorite songs, grabbing your headphones, and making your protein shake. Going to the gym is not actually the ritual, but all the prep elements are, and as you start going through them, it gets less and less likely that you are going to miss your workout. The ritual allows your brain and body the time to slowly start accepting the idea that this workout is a real thing, it's going to happen and it's going to be good. This tough phone call is happening. That pretty girl is about to get

spoken to. That handsome hunk is about to be asked how his day is going. Those folks at Harvard are about to receive this super-bad (which means good) application. It's ON, ladies and gentlemen. The key to a good ritual is that it takes away the decision-making process. When should I do this, how should I do this? What should I do first? Remember that one of the toughest parts in getting going for most people is not really being sure how to get going. Rituals take care of this by making it EASY and AUTOMATIC to get going.

4. **Be very creative when formulating a habit or a ritual:** Most of us are simply not good enough at problem solving when it comes to building their habits and routines and are not ready to reach far enough into the WEIRD category in order to actually get things done. We are often trapped by the paradigms of what we SHOULD be doing, like going to bed at a reasonable hour, or eat certain number of square meals per day. Breaking out of those and establishing habits that actually work, whether that means you set an alarm for 3:00 am, or go stay at the grandparents for a month during exams. Put a handful of almonds in your pocket and take one out every time you reach a goal for the day. Make sure to go home with no almonds left. There are a million creative things you can do to get through the actions that bring your dream to life, just remember that the key is action, and you taking it, consistently.

a) 8-time consecutive Mr. Olympia champion, Ronnie Coleman, gets up at 4:00 am every morning to train, even now that his career is over.

b) Nelson Mandela used to have an ice-cold shower at 5:00 am in prison. Starting his day with something really tough set him up to endure another tough day without his freedom.

c) Maya Angelou rented a local hotel room and went there to write from 6:30 am until 2:00 pm. She never actually spent the night there, but she was able to get her work done.

d) Ivan Lendl, the tennis great, used the same mixtape with the same songs on it for years. The songs and sequence became a part of his habit and routine for getting his mind into the right competitive gear for playing his best tennis.

THE MIDDLE

Now that you have started, are in motion, and have started to build your habit, you are off to a good start. But of course, motivation is a very fickle emotion and can come and go with very little warning. The fact is that most really awesome achievements take a long time, and this means you need to hold your action and motivation state for more than a few weeks. Year 5 of medical school can start to be a drag. Month 4 of the diet can see motivation slipping. The first signs of plateauing can lead to old habits creeping back in. In order to keep going until the deal is done, we need to have a good set of skills to get back on track and not do too much regression damage. Here are some of the secrets to maintaining elite level motivation.

Eliminate potential stressors.

It has been studied and found that the average person responds with an increase in brain wave activity when stress is introduced, yet some elite athletes have a reverse of this phenomenon, they go into a lower brain wave situation, almost a state of meditation. IF you have ever heard a sentence that seems really out of place like "I love the stress, I enjoy it!" from someone and wondered what on earth they are talking about, chances are they are not lying and trying to upset you, but they really do enjoy the stress because it alters their state positively. Obviously, if you do go to a more peaceful state when stressed, then it probably really is enjoyable. For most of us, stress triggers our coping mechanisms. To others, stress IS the coping mechanism. If you are a mere mortal, however, you will most likely respond to stress by, well..., getting stressed out! So, for the vast majority of us, the key is to eliminate potential stressors. Get your homework done, get your presentation sorted, book your tickets, get your ducks in a row. The less you need to worry about on game day, the easier it is to focus and execute. The famous saying that the hardest working employees and top performers always find a way to get things done, while the lowest performing ones are always "too busy" to take on more work is absolutely true. Generally, people who are capable of a lot of high-quality work are good at clearing the clutter, organizing their day and sorting it out.

Learn to talk yourself onto the podium or off the cliff.

Positive self-talk and affirmations go hand in hand, communication with yourself is a vital part of getting through the tough times. People who are self-coaching, "don't let the guy who cut you off get you down, relax a little, you got this, be strong. Fight harder now." Talking to yourself is a wonderful way to remain front-brained and not let the emotions take over, and it has a wonderful benefit of becoming a habit or ritual that can trigger excellent mental discipline. Remember to be conscious and front brained enough to actually realize how you are responding to the stress.

Frame losing correctly in your head.

There are some great sayings out there,

"I never lose, I only win or learn"

"I either win or get great research"

If you want to do anything even remotely cool in this world, you will lose. The cooler the thing you are doing- the more chance your losses will be enormous. You have to make mistakes. You have to have those moments where you bugger things up quite properly. It is quite remarkable to me how many people start a journey and do not have a plan for what will happen when they lose. I hear of some people saying that they never ever think of it, they never plan for it, because this helps them get in the mindset that they have no room for failure. I think this is asinine. You should know that you are very well prepared, have an excellent process and trust your internal and external execution. You should also know that you have an excellent way of dealing with losses and framing them, so that they become the necessary and healthy learning tools that they really are.

Gravity does not lie, and the scoreboard does not either. Knowing this means that the scoreboard is telling you something is missing when you lost. Some decisions, some execution, some planning, some reaction was not quite right, and if you go and find it, you can alter that outcome. I do not believe that winners are good at losing. They tantrum, they moan, they have to work really hard at not losing control of their emotions. What I am saying, is that they are VERY GOOD at assimilating all the necessary information from those losses and feeding it into the computer and coming out with a win the next time around. They do not stay in the loser's circle long. Because of this, they can hold onto their motivation. If you know that your loss angered the heck out of you, and because of this you have been up every day at 5:00 am, training harder than you have in six months, you have made difficult but necessary changes to your game. You are motivated, almost excited to try again. Reason: You reacted well and letting this loss fire you up allowed you to come back to competition motivated. People who make excuses, and make no adjustments to their training, have no reason to believe anything will be different this next time. This means the upcoming competition is daunting, frightening, and most likely will be unenjoyable.

Nurture and feed positive Spirals.

We need to understand spirals. A spiral happens when you start getting a domino effect. You start a diet, you start to lose weight, this gives you great feeling of satisfaction, so you call a friend and go out, and have the confidence to talk to that interesting person you might have been too shy to before you started the diet. Suddenly you are in a relationship, and boom, the rest is history. This can happen just as easily on the flipside. This same relationship is on the rocks, the stress makes you feel bad and you turn to food for comfort. Suddenly, you start gaining weight and in order to combat the guilt and self-loathing from picking the weight back up, you seek comfort in more food. Suddenly you are caught in a negative cycle. They tend to sneak up on you too. When you are winning and being promoted, things are going well it seems like it will last forever. When you are in a negative rut, these too can seem to last a long time. We have to be extremely careful to make sure that the negative spirals don't become a habit. It's quite easy to get comfortable with the idea of mediocrity, and to settle for way less than you are actually capable of or deserve

Anyone who starts doing something will inevitably have some success. A lucky break, the culmination of months of hard work, a better than expected outcome, can all be the triggers that set a really awesome positive cycle in motion. We all know that those cycles can and eventually do come to an end, and we will inevitably have some stops thrown in there along the way. Whether your company shuts down, you get downsized, another stock market meltdown happens, there are a million things that can end a cycle. So, when you get in a really good one, make sure to nurture and feed it and make it last as long as possible.

Avoid the settling cycle.

I have seen many people start out on a mission and start getting some results. It's working, their plan is producing their desired outcome. But then, they get comfortable. Who is going to tell the guy that was top 200 in the world in his sport of expertise that has climbed all the way to 100 that he is settling too soon? We see this time and again, people who had a meteoric rise in the beginning, suddenly settle right as they are arriving on the scene. What changes is their motivation. Think of the kid who comes from a broken home who trains like crazy to escape his chaotic life. He then gets drafted into the NFL, only to become a marginal player. His main motivation was to get out of the house and away from a desperate situation. So with this goal achieved, he does not really have that much motivation to maximize his potential, and undergoes a shift in his internal motivational structure. You need to understand that your motivation is not a static thing, and that you will need to change it from time to time. Think of yourself as a car that runs on multi-fuel. You work with gasoline, electric and diesel. And some days, diesel works just fine, and other days, you need to switch to electric. The top performers are keenly aware that they are not always equally motivated by the same things, and so they have a couple of different motivational sources and have learned that when one fuel source is done and spent, they throw it off like a rocket and switch to some new tanks. It's easy to settle. It's easy to justify settling the higher up the ladder you are.

Break out of negative cycles fast.

Negative cycles can sneak up on you quickly. Suddenly one loss turns into 4. Suddenly 5 pounds turns into 20. Suddenly your routines are not working, you are not feeling the love and you have entered a negative spiral. These bad boys can last for years. Just as excellent thinking can become a habit, so can poor thinking and decision-making. The classic example of the dieter who is amped up, starts strong, then loses their way and quits, feels really guilty and negative and loses their trust in themselves, and ends up 20 pounds heavier than when they started. Negative cycle at its finest. You have to get back to positive action and positive behavior as fast as possible.

Stay in the habitable zone.

Maintaining motivation over a longer time period requires an understanding of how much time you need at the easier level and how much time at the tougher level. When scientists are looking for new earth like planets, they are looking for planets that have specific conditions. One of those is that the distance is not too close or too far from that system's sun. Too close and you burn up all the water and it becomes a wasteland. Too far and it's too cold for liquid water. This distance between too close and too far from the sun is known as the habitable zone. We all have our own motivational habitable zone. If the goals are too tough, we lose motivation, if they are too easy, we also lose motivation. We need to tinker with the formula a little until we find the right mix that keeps us thriving.

If you play tennis against a 4-year-old, you will be too easy, if you play Pete Sampras it will be too hard. Someone closer to your skill level will be more challenging, but sometimes you need a little time in the too hard category, or a little more in the too easy category.

Put your feelings on the shelf.

"I feel tired."

"We had a good week last week."

"It's ok to take a little break."

"The weather is not great."

Those are feelings. Those need to go up on the shelf. Discipline is the thing that manages the incredibly creative human excuse machine. It's actually remarkable that we are not all top executive salesmen, because we have been able to sell ourselves on some of the most amazing excuses over our lives!

"He is too good for me,"

"I am not smart enough,"

"We are not hurting anyone,"

FINISH

It's important to understand an interesting mechanism when it comes to completing a task. You might experience a reversal of motivation. Your body likes your routine and has gotten used to it, and has figured out the daily grind, and now suddenly your book, or movie, or degree is coming to an end. Your mind knows there is going to be a huge void when you are done. Buyer's remorse the day after you get the Maserati is a little bit the same phenomenon. Self-sabotage can kick in. A great way to get good at finishing things is to have your next adventure planned already.

Anticipation: The best in just about anything have developed the skill of anticipating. They spend a lot less time reacting to things than most people, and far more time being proactive. Anticipate that your motivation will drop, change and need to be managed, and have a plan to do just that. Motivation at a deeper level. We have some deeper motivations at play, and we need to talk about how those affect us on a daily basis. We start with what we call the success bias, and how a motivation to succeed differs from a motivation to avoid failure.

Motivation to succeed: These are people who gather their resources and excitement when there is a perceived opportunity ahead of them. They feel that if they work their tails off, they can achieve the thing they have their mind set on.

People who are motivated by success don't need as much instruction or cajoling when the chips are down, things are not going well—they see it as an opportunity to turn things around and be heroes.

Motivation to Avoid Failure:

Generally described as someone who responds to something that challenges their EGO. They desperately do not want to be humiliated. Their confidence is linked to the difficulty of the situation- if it's perceived to be easy, confidence is high, if it's perceived to be difficult, confidence drops. However, people whose focus is on avoiding failure generally need direction. They need to be told what to do so they'll feel they can react correctly when backed into a corner. (Otherwise, they'll be convinced they don't have a chance.) Take your average football game, for example. One team is up by two points in the closing seconds of the game. The opposing team has the ball and has just crossed midfield. A good coach or quarterback needs to tell the players who are most likely to focus on failure exactly what to do, in this case to cover their territory while in a zone defense or just use their footwork during pass coverage. This kind of instruction removes some of the self-induced pressure from a person, allowing him to focus on the task at hand.

Generally, the motivation to go to your job, even though you don't like it could be described as motivation to avoid failure. You have to go, you don't want to lose your house, you need the money, you have bills to pay. This is not part of some masterplan to succeed, this is you doing just what you need to sustain your current lifestyle. I have met hundreds of people who will get out of bed and go do something they really don't like for decades, because the motivation to avoid failure is so strong. These same people will always tell you they can't or don't have time to start working on their dream and the lifestyle they really do want. The two most common excuses are always too tired or too busy. At some level they don't believe it's actually possible, or that they deserve it, and so they settle for just chugging along and avoiding the failure of getting the house repossessed, rather than take some risk and go after a lifestyle they REALLY DO want.

Show UP.

Lives are permanently and magically transformed by this one simple step. You decided to show up to show up to something that mattered to you. The common mistake here, however, is that most people wait to show up because their inward feeling is that they are not ready or prepared enough to present themselves to a new audience. If they would just go and show up - regardless of how they felt about their outward appearance, diet, or level of education, they'd be astounded to see that the group they're showing up for is not much better than themselves. In fact, they might learn that they are an asset, someone that can offer a great deal to others. When we speak about our own imagination of what is needed, or what the great superstars have that we don't, we essentially talk ourselves out of so many things. When I was younger and was training in the same academy as the number one player in the country at the time, I saw firsthand how he lived on a daily basis. I saw the laziness, the tantrums, the average choices, and the middle of the road stuff. I immediately thought that he was good, but also human, and that I was capable of at least copying his habits, and possibly even going one step better than them.

The UTILITY of your goal.

Imagine for a moment that you are a soul floating around in outer space. You are looking for a vehicle to live out an incredible experience, and so you start to flip through space-Google, looking for a human body to rent for 80-90 years. Renting this machine would allow you to express all your love, passions, hopes, dreams, have fun. IF you compare what it would cost to rent a private plane all day every day for 80 years, you could imagine the cost of a human body would be immense. Let's say for argument's sake, it costs you $500k per month. That's $6 mil a year. Now you dedicate yourself with full power for 5 years towards the goal of getting a Maserati, worth $150k. You have spent $30,000,000 on chasing something worth only a fraction of that. I am not here to tell you what to chase or not chase, but if you are having a hard time getting motivated for something you think you want, you might be running into a problem with the utility of your goals. Setting your ship to a higher purpose often feels way better and allows us to tap into motivation more easily.

CHAPTER 8: DISCIPLINE

D
iscipline is a word that needs to hire a good PR agent. Most people I meet are taken aback when I tell them we are going to make their lives more disciplined. They get the image of waking up in Siberia, with some 300 pound military drill sergeant named Vladimir telling them to "pliz crank wan hundred pushes" They think of missing important social events as they are holed up in their rooms, studying for their millionth test. They imagine a world of having to give up things, vacant of all the juice and spice that makes things fun and entertaining, and the solitude of the hard-daily grind being their only companion.

The reality is actually very different. Discipline when well-developed is the ultimate tool of self-expression. It is a choice between indulging in activities that mute development or managing your time and resources in such a way that you are able to more fully express a value or idea. One of my favorite examples to begin with is the great horror novelist, Stephen King. He is known for writing at the same time, for the exact same amount of time, every day. He wakes up, sits down, and works on his writing. He admits that a lot of what he writes is not usable, but, as we know, he has written 88 books, 34 of which have been made into movies. Considering this book has taken me almost 2 years to write, I would need to live 190 years to equal this feat!

Discipline actually equals having more fun. It equals having more sustained fun. If we think about what we are most

disciplined about, it's most probably our jobs. We show up every day, and we most definitely fear the consequence of getting fired if we don't show up often enough. "The punishment" for not showing up is real, it's severe, so we end up being pretty disciplined. We show up every day. But when it comes to our dreams, and doing the stuff we really want to do, we often put it off and display all the characteristics of not having discipline. How often do you see the hardworking couple that puts off going on vacation, puts off doing the cruise for later? Instead of a disciplined savings plan that enables them to do these things and be fine, they put them off and waste the money of silly mall trips, millions of Starbucks coffees, and experiences that are not enriching at all.

Discipline is the most remarkable enabler of skill and lifestyle. You think about the lifestyle of a professional athlete. Arriving at a beautiful stadium court is fantastic, exhilarating, overwhelming and magnificent, all at the same time. Flying to different cities, countries, locations is a freedom most people will never have. But it does not end there. The rewards allow them to have beautiful things, comfortable homes, nice cars. And still, it does not end there, they have bodies that are in beautiful shape, healthy and vibrant, full of energy.

The discipline, the hard stuff actually makes life such an incredible experience. Most of us start from the viewpoint that being a champion will never happen for us, we tend to take the attitude of "this cake does not matter, this Netflix marathon doesn't really make a difference." The classic idea of viewing the glass as half full or viewing it as half empty really does find a home here. If you view discipline through the 'half-empty' lens of what you will be giving up, it will feel more difficult, and motivation might be an issue. If you view it through the 'half-full' perspective of what you will be gaining, you will most likely find it much easier to follow through.

Very few of us have ever experienced what sustained discipline can do for our lives. We have no relationship to what owning a private jet or owning a villa in the south of Spain is like. We most definitely do not link these things to the idea of discipline. We have never earned them, nor have we existed in a sustained state of discipline for long enough to understand that these rewards were the result of that process. Instead we think of how hungry we will be right now if we give up on the cake, how lonely we will be tonight if we don't go out for drinks. What will our friends say about us if we are not there?

Top performers know the secret of discipline. Once something is ingrained to the level of habit, it becomes a lifestyle. This means that you don't have to actually fight through the negative feelings and inertia to get started. It's not actually as difficult as most people think it is to get going and keep going.

Let's take a look at some of the essentials of good discipline:

1. THE 'IN-SPITE-OF' RULE

This little magic trick relies on mental sleight-of-hand. The first thing a good surgeon will recommend when there is a blockage, is to do a bypass. Reroute the blood around the blockage. The 'In-Spite-Of' rule works in much the same way. Think of it as a brain bypass.

"I am tired and cranky, but IN SPITE OF that, I'll practice anyway."

"I won the tournament last week and I am feeling like spoiling myself with a day off, but IN SPITE OF that, I'll practice today anyway."

No matter what the attempted excuse is, you have to use this little piece of mental bypass surgery to get around the blockage. Here is a great example from one of the all-time great skateboarders, Tony Hawk. Here he is talking about a new spiral ramp with extreme difficulty. Pay attention to how he uses the IN SPITE OF technique.

"I must be honest, when I realized this project got the green light, that Sony is behind it, I had intense anxiety for 2 days. I couldn't stop thinking about it. Is it real? Will it work? I have no idea what to expect. I am worried about not sticking to the wall, or having no control coming out the bottom and shooting off uncontrollably. There is going to be a lot of energy in such a tight space…and it has to go somewhere. If I let the anxiety take over, then it's going to be worst case scenario, because that's all I have thought about. I DO think it's possible, and that I AM capable of doing it. That's what I am going to hold onto."

Just a great example of working through the feelings, the anxiety, but then saying, in spite of all the million feelings and reasons why my brain is creating to get me to not do this, I am going to focus on just two empowering thoughts:

1. It is possible

2. I am capable of doing it.

Those two thoughts are all you need to make you act.

DISCIPLINE IS THE MOTHER OF CREATIVITY.

I remember when I was young thinking, how does doing the same thing over and over, having routines, how does this help you be creative? If there was ever anything like hidden dimensions, then discipline gives you the keys to access them. I was a small-town kid from a semi-podunk city that was not exactly known for producing professional athletes. It wasn't particularly good at producing stellar students either. It was pretty good at producing middle-of-the-road.

When I was 12, I was playing a lot of tennis, but there is no way I could have imagined that 7 years later, I would be playing in the main draw at a Grand Slam tournament. There is no way I could imagine where I would find the funding, how I would travel to the tournaments, and make it happen. If I had focused on those questions, then I would have gotten really anxious and fallen apart. So, I just focused on the tennis. The other stuff happened, as if by magic, as if by some quantum entanglement, my desire and work ethic called out to the universe and it waved its magic wand for me.

I was suddenly opening a locker in Australia, Pete Sampras right next door. How on earth is something like this possible?

Somewhere, whether it is hour 250 or 4,000 of your 10,000 hours developing yourself into an expert, you are going to have multiple breakthroughs. You can never predict when or how, but they happen giving birth to huge amounts of skill. You learn and your skill set grows. You will be doing new, more complicated things soon in your routine. Let's think about math at school. We all remember doing a million multiplication tables. Then we got pretty good at it, and we ended up going to the next progressions: division, fractions and so forth. Pretty soon you are quite competent, and you are doing things that humans just 50 years ago had not even invented yet. This is how it goes when you become a highly disciplined person. By making the time to do the thing that you want and building that habit and routine, you open yourself up to the progressions that are available.

Travel the world. Meet amazing people. Do something at a level that is awesome. Inspire and engage with the young and the dreamers and make sure to leave them with a warm and incredible experience. These things are all much better than watching Netflix. Touring a museum, seeing the best art ever made, standing dumbfounded in front of some of the world's most incredible architecture. These things are all much better than wobbling down the steps in your wife-beater vest, and having a 4000-calorie butter, egg, syrup and bacon bomb.

Ok, so everyone in the world, barring a small percentage, would like to be more disciplined. Let's figure out a way to get there. What are the key ingredients to developing good discipline? Developing self-discipline is the crucible of success,

According to a 2013 study by Wilhelm Hoffman, people with high self-control are happier than those without. The study discovered this is true because the self-disciplined subjects were more capable of dealing with goal conflicts. These people spent less time debating whether to indulge in behaviors detrimental to their health and were able to make positive decisions more easily. The self-disciplined did not allow their choices to be dictated by impulses or feelings. Instead, they made informed, rational decisions on a daily basis without feeling overly stressed or upset.

Plan the stuff you need to be disciplined about. Make sure you actually know what it is you need to do and when you need to do it. This seems pretty logical and simple, but realistically, so many people start their week without a plan that they are in that reactive, 'life is happening to me' state. You need to know when you are going to the gym, what you are eating, when you are buying those groceries, when you are working, what social events you have planned. And when your vices will be enjoyed.

1. Wait…. What..? He said Vices? Yes. Work hard play hard. If you plan the rewards in ahead of time, and you know you have something to look forward to, you can easily push through one or two of the tough days, knowing your payday is coming soon.

You do not need to be vice free to be disciplined. In fact, most of the people I know who are really disciplined, have learned how to let loose the right way. Funny enough, if you think about it in terms of nutrition, is actually good for your metabolism to throw in a high calorie day from time to time.

Have fun nurturing and developing your vice, something you are willing to go the extra mile for (side note, let's try and stick to weekends at the cabin, travel, a pizza or ice cream, maybe some gaming on the PlayStation here, and not a repeat of the movie, The Hangover!)

1. This brings us to number 3. Since being disciplined is hard enough as it is, it does not help to have majorly clashing priorities, vices that require 4 days to recover

from, things that trigger so much stress and so many coping mechanisms that they pull you away from being able to focus on being disciplined. So, try and clear away the clutter. Try to simplify your life as much as possible. As with any well lived life, there is a tendency to want to take it all in, but if you want to become disciplined, you will need to sit down and make some decisions on what to cut, how to trim the fat to make this a lean and tasty life-steak.

2. Anxiety is not your friend. Food is probably the most abused drug for anxiety and stress, and exercise is the most underused antidepressant. When you get super anxious, your discipline is going to go out the window. Excess anxiety will occupy prime real estate in your mind and become the thing that you are thinking about the most. It can push you to become a primal, manic state. Discipline has vanished like water vapor from a kettle. Converting water into steam is one thing, converting it from steam back to water is the tricky part!

3. David Copperfield stuff is an illusion: The world tends to want magic tricks. It tends to want quick answers. It tends to want fairy tales. We put great achievers on a pedestal as if they are some great mythical creature. I can assure you, they are no different than any other person. They got lucky to be able to find an environment that allowed them to work for many hours at a skill set. This means they got good. Period. There is no Santa Claus, and there is no mythical talent button. You have one of the most highly sophisticated machines in the universe at your disposal, the human body. Don't kid yourself. This thing is unbelievably

capable, and its purpose built to go and test those capabilities. Holding yourself back is a total waste and being scared of the competition is also a waste. So, let's take some folks off the pedestal, and let's train and prepare very well, and let's see just how good they actually are.

2. The 10 000-hour promise.

You are not going to become good enough at anything to seriously move the needle in your life without putting in the right amount of time developing your skill. Please, for the love of Pete, don't give up on yourself before this number. So many people have actually made amazing progress by 3000 hours, but they feel like they should be getting the results that someone with 8000 hours should be getting and so they become deactivated and quit. Be realistic, know where you are at, and promise to stay the course.

1. The "master craftsman, whose time has come." This is when you have been training for years, working, eating the failures, being right up against the quitting line and persevering when there was absolutely no good reason to do so. Very few people will ever know what the other side of this part of being disciplined feels like, they just don't master their craft enough. For those who do stay the course, and are willing to work through the tough times, hanging onto their dream like someone hanging onto a rope tied to the back of a car and being dragged through the streets. But they take

the bruises, take the nicks and cuts and scratches and finally they arrive at the opening of a huge opportunity. Something that changes their lives, permanently.

They get the BIG REWARD.

CHAPTER 9: LEARNING

The story of learning is about utility. Anyone with two hands and two feet can shovel snow. You can shovel snow for 8 dollars an hour for a thousand years and still not become a millionaire. If you want to go up in the world, you need to add utility. This means you need to be more useful to more people. Bill Gates' company, Microsoft has enormous utility, billions of computers worldwide rely on the Windows operating system to function. Steve Jobs mounted his comeback at Apple based on the premise of utility. He offered millions an easy way to store and listen to their songs, thousands of them, from a little device that fits in your pocket.

Utility. It's as big a word as any in the successful person's dictionary. Jeff Bezos has built Amazon around utility. Millions of us rely on his company to get things we could never get before, quicker, more seamlessly and at a fraction of their former cost. Serving a billion people a day: that is the very definition of utility. The question is quite simply, how many people you are helping through your skill set, how often, and how replaceable are you. If you are a top neurosurgeon, you have monumental utility to the person who just came in from the car accident. If you clean someone's house, unfortunately you have a fairly low utility.

AI MACHINE LEARNING.

Ok, o you recognize that your skill set does not offer a lot of solutions people are desperate for, and you are hellbent on changing this. The good news for you is that you have one of

the most advanced learning machines in the universe at your disposal, this insane piece of biological equipment called the human body (my attitude on the incredible capabilities of the human body is not a secret at this point!)

How does learning work exactly? Learning is actually quite simple. We need a pretty big data set. The 10 000-hour rule is a decent starting point. Rome was not built in a day, and you have very little chance of becoming a world beater without putting in the requisite time and pain and suffering. The next thing you need is a way to analyze and process the data from your attempts. Each next attempt needs to build on the previous one, gradually ironing out the wrinkles and paving the way for progress.

We can actually learn a lot about learning from computers. Computers have come a long way over the last two decades, and the results of their capacity to "learn" are perhaps best displayed in two very difficult skills they have now permanently surpassed humans in, Chess and Go

Deep Blue became famous around the world when it beat the world's best ever chess player, Gary Kasparov. For those not familiar with the dominance of the Russian grandmaster, he played professionally from 1986 to 2005 and held the world number 1 spot for a staggering 225 months. So, he was pretty good.

It was no surprise then, that a little ripple of terror flew through the hearts and minds of the people as one of the deep intellectual super minds of our time fell to a machine for the first time in 1997. Deep Blue, a computer program built by IBM, beat the unbeatable.

The only game left that humans had the upper hand on was the ancient Chinese game of Go, which, although it has more simple rules, offers a far deeper and more complex logic tree. Simply put, it has more possible moves with each turn, which correlates to millions more possible move combinations and some extreme computing power to calculate them.

Ladies and gentlemen, to the left of the arena, please enter Lee Sodol. And to the right, from the folks at Google DeepMind, please enter AlphaGo. A brilliant 5 match series to watch, there was an incredible moment called the 'GOD MOVE' by Lee Sodol, where he came up with a move that no computer, including AlphaGo could predict, even with its monumental computing power. A true testimony to the enormity of the power of the human brain. That being said, the computer won the series 4-1, and marked the beginning of a new era in computers, the era of machine learning.

Of course, we are not really that worried about the rise of terminator machines: huge muscled, red-eyed, flesh covered titanium alloy with thick Austrian accents sent back in time to destroy us. Instead, what we want to know is the HOW part of the way these computers acquired their skill. While human achievement has been shrouded in secrecy and washed over with words like talent, genetic ability, etc., these computers had a zero-starting point before being taught how to beat the world's best. They did not need talent. They did not need genes. They did not need boatloads of self-confidence.

So, how exactly did we teach machines to be smarter than ourselves? Here is what the makers of AlphaGo say: "AlphaGo and its successors use a Monte Carlo tree search algorithm to find its moves based on knowledge previously "learned" by machine learning, specifically by an artificial neural network (a deep learning method) by extensive training, both from human and computer play." In other words, the machine did its homework. It studied really hard, and it completed a colossal amount of trial and error in match-play both simulated and real time, against actual and imaginary opponents.

Wait.

Isn't this how we also get good?

The cat is out of the bag. The most monumental achievements are attainable by following this simple method. It is pretty obvious that humans will lose, and lose badly, to machines in all of these types of endeavors, because we simply can never work through as big of a data set as a computer, but you certainly can work through a bigger data set than your fellow man. You just need to stay emotionally primed to do this.

Where the computer has a big advantage over us (apart from not needing sleep, food, having to stop to take kids to school) etc., is that it is phlegmatic to failure. It's not afraid to look ridiculous a few hundred thousand times.

We often get caught up in an emotional response to improvement. Have a look at an example of poor human feedback below:

"I look like a spaz right now"

"What if I spend all this time and I still don't improve"

"What other things could I be doing right now"

"Grrr, this is making me really frustrated."

Now compare this with the computer. Its program simply states the computer will run 100 attempts today. Of those 100 it will start with attempt number 67 from yesterday again, as this attempt was the closest to success. It will be making x and y modifications to number 67 and running from there.

Computer: Run number 67 with x and y modifications.

Result: x modification was helpful,

y modification, unhelpful.

Discard y and exchange for z modification

Run again

Undisturbed by human needs, the computer has free reign to harness the power of progress versus regress, and by holding on to progress, will be able to continue learning.

As we distill this down to our own use, we know for a fact that all humans are capable of a monumental level of growth and learning, provided we have a couple of key ingredients.

1. Large enough sample set. Commit mentally for years, not months or weeks.

2. Fail, make modifications, fail again. Fail better. Fail towards success. Generally, good teachers will suggest your modifications, but many greats simultaneously develop a system of self-improvement where they decide the modifications for themselves.

3. Jump to your next progression at the right time: It can be tricky mastering the   balance between discipline and creativity. As a general rule, we need to perform a task until close to perfection and at this point, we need to add complexity to the task and again seek mastery. It can take an extreme amount of engagement, focus, and raw creativity to search for and find the next evolutionary progression but search for progressions we must if we are to adapt and grow. Try to progress too soon and you end up with a different type of dilemma. Each concept builds on the former concept, and also serves as a foundation for the next level. If you try to jump ahead too soon, you end up mired in difficulty because there is a gap of knowledge and skill.

TIME, RESOURCES, 10,000 HOURS AND THE ECONOMICS OF BEING A GROWN UP.

One of the biggest hurdles to building a higher utility, higher functioning you is that you need to expose yourself to the huge data set that facilitates the learning process. This needs to happen in conjunction with work, kids, working out, family, birthdays, out of town friends, travel and the myriad of other things that make up the modern lifestyle. It needs surplus funds, or the capacity to function on a lower budget for a while.

Changing fields and learning a new trade is not an easy task. The most important thing to remember is that you are trying to replace a 10 000-hour, low utility but still polished skill set, with one that is higher utility, but still only at 1,000 hours. This means you are going to have to do both for the foreseeable future. You need to ply your trade in order to pay the bills and keep the ship sailing, while at the same time putting in your 10,000 hours to bring the new skill up to speed.

It is for this very reason that most people can't see a clear path to actually skill-up or change their career path. Carrying 2 major projects at the same time is a daunting and severe lifestyle for a while. But of course, it can be done, and it has been done many times with the right mindset and support.

A LIFESTYLE OF LEARNING, THE MODERN-DAY RENAISSANCE MAN.

Most of us are done with learning when we graduate from college. After this, we head into the work field and start to apply our trade. Yes, we most certainly do learn critical, on-the-job nuances, but as far as learning a new skill set altogether, we generally do not. I like to think back to the times of Leonardo Da Vinci and Michelangelo, guys who were trained in multiple disciplines such as architecture, engineering, art, languages and they probably could turn on a lightbulb just by blinking.

There was a culture in that time that celebrated the learning skills of humanity, and the art of being accomplished. I fear the pressures of modern society have perhaps eroded this mind-set. Perhaps, the legendary Carl Sagan says it best,

"I have a foreboding of an America in my children's or grandchildren's time -- when the United States is a service and information economy; when nearly all the manufacturing industries have slipped away to other countries; when awesome technological powers are in the hands of a very few, and no one representing the public interest can even grasp the issues; when the people have lost the ability to set their own agendas or knowledgeably question those in authority; when, clutching our crystals and nervously consulting our horoscopes, our critical faculties in

decline, unable to distinguish between what feels good and what's true, we slide, almost without noticing, back into superstition and darkness...

The dumbing down of America is most evident in the slow decay of substantive content in the enormously influential media, the 30 second sound bites (now down to 10 seconds or less), lowest common denominator programming, credulous presentations on pseudoscience and superstition, but especially a kind of celebration of ignorance"

CARL SAGAN

Ok. So, you are a modern-day renaissance-millennial. You are in. Sold. Higher utility is for you. You want to skill up and open new doors of opportunity for yourself and your family. You are ready to expose yourself to the stresses and logistics challenges of getting in your 10 ,00 hours.

Good for you. The last step is to understand and recognize your learning style. Let's quickly go through them and then we are off to the races. There are 8 basic learning styles, and chances are you are a combination of some of the ones below, but have one that sticks out as your primary human machine learning mega intake method:

The Linguistic Learner.

This type of learning style learns best through reading, writing, listening and speaking skills. Read about your subject matter, listen to an audiobook, take some notes. Find a group to talk about it or write articles on your subject matter.

The Environmental Learner.

Being out in the field, interacting with the world around you, being out in nature. This type of person learns best doing experiments and being very hands on in the great outdoors. The experience and freedom of being able to move through open spaces, possibly not have too many people around. A nice example is Albert Einstein who always did his best thinking on his long outdoor walks through nature.

The Musical, Rhythm Based Learner.

The obvious one here is a musician who learns to put notes together in interesting ways. There is also the person who learns better with background noise, humming, toe tapping, music in the background. Try this next time you hit the books to see if you have some musical learning chemistry! You might find you do your best thinking with some sounds in the background.

The Kinesthetic Learner.

Hands on. Gotta feel it. Gotta actually take the bull by the horns and ride it to learn. This type of person gravitates towards hands on careers. Physical therapist, sports person, plumber, construction and surgeon are all fields a kinesthetic learner would find comfortable.

The Visual or Spatial Learner

We take in an enormous amount of information through our eyes. Contrast the amount of times you used your eyes in order to learn, versus the number of times you used smell or even hearing to learn. Diagrams, pictures, graphs, and videos are all examples of visual training aids. Spatial skills encompass being able to work on conceptual projects, for example the insides of a computer without actually ever seeing them. Architects, 3D CAD, sculpting all require the spatial understanding element.

The Logic/Math Based Learner

If you like computing numbers, finding relationships between data sets, analyzing the strategies of your favorite NFL team, finding logical reasons for the world around you, then you are a math-based person. Scientists, engineers, Nasa applicants, please step forward.

The Interpersonal Learner

We have all had that one teacher who made a profound impact on our lives. The connection with someone who made you excel at a way faster pace that you otherwise would have. We normally elevate this person to the level of Mentor, as the amount of exposure and understanding of new ideas under their tutelage far surpassed any other person we have encountered. The reality is this was an example of an awesome interpersonal teacher-student experience. If you work well with mentors, seek out and find the best experts you can find, consistently.

The Intrapersonal Learner

As we go through these 8 learning styles, I am sure you have a sense that you are a combination of these. The intrapersonal learner likes to do the bulk of the learning by themselves, they like solving problems on their own time and with their own agenda. They work best in jobs with no direct supervision, so we are thinking Sales, Entrepreneur, Writer here.

WHERE DO WE GET OUR KNOWLEDGE?

This is an incredibly important idea: where and how do we get our knowledge. Google has been a tremendous invention as it has redefined freedom of information flow and made knowledge much more accessible, to many more people. The great fear with giving knowledge away for free has been that the people who controlled this knowledge will lose the advantage they have, and this could lead to loss of income and earnings. As we have seen, this is rarely the case. Cars have been around for nearly 100 years, but very few of us have taken the time to figure out how the engines work, or how to build one. Bottom line, even if you give people the same ingredients, it is unlikely that they will bake the same type of cake. Which means your particular way of baking it is safe for the most part.

It is critical for the future that we are building populations that are as educated as possible. Making education and access to it easier has to be the next revolution. If you think what Uber has been able to do to the transport industry- there has to be something similar on the horizon for the world of education, and I wouldn't be surprised if we see more big companies following in Elon Musk's footsteps and opening up their patents for everyone to use.

What you DO want is to tap into the enormous number of online courses, great YouTube how to videos, and million other sources out there to get access to the info that going to propel you forward.

What you DON'T want is to spend your 10 000 hours doing the wrong stuff. So, make sure you find your learning style, make sure you have a couple of experts on standby, and make sure you have an idea of what your next progression is going to be, and then get going. A new higher utility, higher opportunity mining you awaits!

Chapter 10: The Dark Hour

My darkest hour was a place I never thought I would get to. I had always been proud of myself and someone who was honest, hard-working, and successful. I had started out my tennis career on a positive note and was a young crusader inside the top 200 in the world. I had always believed that working hard and doing the right things would make you feel incredible inside and would create a world that was beautiful and fun to experience. I believed that the most stressful moments would highlight your core character, and as such, I sought out bigger and bigger challenges, each time convinced it was the beliefs, ideas and values that I nurtured that I could rely on to steady the ship as we hit the rough seas. I absolutely loved what I did and being a professional tennis player was the only thing I could imagine doing for the rest of my life.

POP- the sound that no athlete wants to hear. The knee had been horrible, sore, swollen, uncomfortable. But this was the big daddy. Moments after the pop noise, you actually don't feel that much pain, it's more of a visceral, nauseous feeling at first. The body knows something is up.

The diagnosis came back in as a ruptured patellar tendon, and the procedure was going to be tricky. Take a third of the patella out. The doctors were talking about abstract concepts like quality of life, and good chance you can lead a pretty full and normal life. I remember the information was trying to make its way into my head, my brain was doing its job of deciphering

the underlying meaning of those sentences. My stubbornness was raging, "You guys are clowns, so conservative, always protecting yourself from lawsuits, always giving the lowest common denominator, lowest risk determination. We both know I am going to play again, this is a minor setback"

What followed was the slowest 18 months of my life. I was stuck in some kind of athlete-regular person purgatory, not really sure what the end result would be, still clinging to a dream that I could be a tennis player. Still hanging on to the idea that had been a part of my life for as long as I could remember.

There was always a part of me that fully understood the luxury of self-expression. I don't think for one minute of my tennis career I was not keenly aware of the very few people globally who find their passion or find an avenue of self-expression that is both challenging and fulfilling. I knew how fortunate I was to be a tennis player. I fought as hard as I could for anything in my life. I was not ready to give up the dream. I was not ready to give up my art form.

18 months after surgery, I played my first professional tennis match again. Something was different, I couldn't move as well as I wanted to, and I knew that I could never reach the heights I had seen in my mind. I learned something important about the sheer bliss of chasing the next big idea, the next evolutionary progression. What is next? What does 1 percent better look like? Feel Like? What training methods are needed to find it?

Before the injury, it was this incredible exhilarating and consuming game, and I was a young master that the world better look out for....

After my comeback, I was playing, winning here and there, but not really improving, and because of my physical limitations, arriving at tournaments under prepared and definitely not enthusiastic and chasing brilliance. I was lost. Playing because I did not know what else to do. I was not playing well or training well because my body wouldn't let me.

It's Five a.m. I haven't slept at all. Trying to numb the pain in my leg had meant taking painkillers by the fistful. I am trying to drown out the noise in my head- I have probably pissed off or alienated every person on earth that's tried to comfort or help me. I am completely broken inside.

I decide to go for a run- high on painkillers- middle of nowhere.

I want to try and explain the feeling I had inside which is that you have this one life, and this one chance to do something really cool, and I have a huge doubt that I will ever find something that I like or want to do as much as I liked tennis. I have lost the most important thing that will ever happen to me. AND IT HURTS. IT'S THE EMOTIONAL EQUIVALENT OF EATING A HOT COAL FROM A FIRE, TRYING TO SWALLOW THIS GLOWING RED-HOT LUMP, AND THEN AFTER THE AGONY OF ACTUALLY SWALLOWING IT, DEALING WITH THE CONSTANT INDIGESTION OF HAVING A GLOWING LUMP OF BURNING COAL IN THE GUT. FABULOUS.

People look at you and wonder why you are not paying full attention, not present. It's hard to see from the outside that you have this GLOWING HOT LUMP OF SOUL-COAL occupying your mind-

And, let's not even go to those special days when a text would come through- "wow, I see a friend of yours _____ (insert name of choice here) has just made semifinals of a grand slam" Watching your peers achieve success after success as you drown in the loss of your career is no fun, and I don't wish it on anyone. That's not to say I don't wish my compadres well, that's not even remotely the point- it is just extremely difficult to watch the world go by and you are suddenly not on the train.

I feel ill. I am running. I am tired. Haven't slept. Don't want to. What I see and feel when I close my eyes is too debilitating, too sad.

I am in deep shit.

I decide to go and see a professional. And honestly, it's the best thing I have ever done. It only took me 2 sessions to let all of that out. To just tell someone how incredibly sad I was at the loss of my number one love. To have someone hear it. Me, the tough guy, brought to his knees. Those dreams as a kid- and the most important one- the dream of holding a coveted trophy had been fueling my existence for years. This story was going to end in an incredible way. It didn't. It ended with a tendon that ruptured.

On the one planet that we know life exists, it is extremely pervasive. If you think about the forces of gravity, electromagnetism, the strong and weak nuclear force as the fundamental forces of nature, we have a fundamental force inside of us that seeks creativity. And when one door to creativity shuts, your body feels extreme emotional pain, because that need to create is so strong. But you can rest assured, while you are burning, your brain and soul are searching for a new way to express. As long as you make absolutely sure that you don't take on any new travelers of the "bad perspective" type and start viewing the world through damaged lens of negative outlook, you will bounce back and have a lot of fun doing it.

As with any bad break up, you are consumed for a while. Then.... sneakily, suddenly...... without warning.... You notice someone new for the first time. Your little damaged soul reaches out like the tiny little green shoot of a vine searching for a new place to take hold.

What you need to know is this. Everyone has their dark hour. Everyone has their toughest, most challenging moments of their lives. Everyone thinks the world has ended and life will never be the same again. But that life-force that pulses so completely within you will not be denied. It will find a way.

CHAPTER 11: BREAKTHROUGH

THE MILLION DOLLAR MACHINE.

All breakthroughs start in your head. We very often hold onto a poor perspective for years, reacting to the ideas and actions that stem from that perspective for years, until finally we evolve into a different one, and are left thinking about what a waste some or all of the energy spent in that mindset was.

Anchoring yourself in a strong perspective can be both incredibly liberating, or it can become an internal prison of sorts. Breakthroughs happen when you have those internal shifts. When you finally arrive at a great perspective.

What is the value of you? If you asked the best scientists at MIT to build an exact replica of you, eyes, ears, smell, decision making, ability to learn, what would that machine cost in research and development costs, then materials and parts?

You are worth a fortune! Millions and millions of dollars! All of our super advanced science has still not found a way to duplicate you-

Sometimes we forget just how insanely lottery-esque it is that we were born in the first place. So, let's go through this wonderful probability exercise by Dr Ali Binazir to wrap our heads around the chances of you being you.

This wonderful piece by Dr. Ali Binazir has always given me a good smile, as well as driven home the point that you are

in fact, EVEN MORE special than your mom used to tell you. This piece is about just how slim the odds

"First, let's talk about the probability of your parents meeting. If they met one new person of the opposite sex every day from age 15 to 40, that would be about 10,000 people. Let's confine the pool of possible people they could meet to 1/10th of the world's population 20 years go (1/10th of 4 billion = 400 million) so it considers not just the population of the US but that of the places they could have visited. Half of those people, or 200 million, will be of the opposite sex. So, let's say the probability of your parents meeting, ever, is 10,000 divided by 200 million, or one in 20,000.

Step 1. Probability of boy meeting girl: one in 20,000.

So far, so good.

Now let's say the chances of them actually *talking* to one another is one in 10. And the chances of that turning into another meeting is about one in 10 also. And the chances of that turning into a long-term relationship is also one in 10. And the chances of *that* lasting long enough to result in offspring is one in two. So, the probability of your parents' chance meeting resulting in kids is about one in 2000.

Step 2. Probability of same boy knocking up same girl: one in 2000.

So, the combined probability is already around one in 40 million — long but not insurmountable odds. Now things start getting interesting. We're about to deal with eggs and sperm, which come in large numbers.

You are the result of the fusion of one particular egg with one particular sperm. Each sperm and each egg are genetically unique because of the process of meiosis. A fertile woman has 100,000 viable eggs on average. A man will produce about 12 trillion sperm over the course of his reproductive lifetime. Let's say a third of those (4 trillion) are relevant to our calculation, since the sperm created after a woman hits menopause don't count. So, the probability of that one sperm with half your name on it hitting that one egg with the other half of your name on it is one in 400 quadrillion.

Step 3. Probability of right sperm meeting right egg: one in 400 quadrillion.

But we're just getting started.

Because the existence of you here now on planet earth presupposes another supremely unlikely and utterly undeniable chain of events. Namely, that *every one of your ancestors lived to reproductive age* — going all the way back not just to the first Homo sapiens, first Homo erectus and Homo habilis, but all the way back to the first single-celled organism. You are a representative of an unbroken lineage of life going back 4 billion years.

Let's not get carried away here; we'll just deal with the human lineage. Say humans or humanoids have been around for about 3 million years, and that a generation is about 20 years. That's 150,000 generations. Say that over the course of all human existence, the likelihood of any one human offspring to survive childhood and live to reproductive age and have at least one kid is 50:50 — one in two. Then what would be the chance of your particular lineage to have remained unbroken for 150,000 generations?

Well then, that would be one in 2,150,000 which is about one in 1045,000 — a number so staggeringly large that my head hurts just writing it down. That number is not just larger than all of the particles in the universe — it's larger than all the particles in the universe if each particle were itself a universe.

Step 4. Probability of every one of your ancestors reproducing successfully: one in 1045,000

But let's think about this some more. Remember the sperm-meeting-egg argument for the creation of you, since each gamete is unique? Well, the right sperm also had to meet the right egg to create your grandparents, too. Otherwise they'd be different people, and so would their children, who would then have had children who were similar to you but not quite you. This is also true of their parents, and so on till the beginning of time. If even once the wrong sperm met the wrong egg, you would not be sitting here noodling online reading fascinating articles like this one. It would be your cousin Jethro, and you never really liked him anyway.

That means in every step of your lineage, the probability of the right sperm meeting the right egg such that the exact right ancestor would be created that would end up creating you is one in 400 quadrillion.

So now we must account for those 150,000 generations by raising 400 quadrillion to the 150,000th power:

$$[4 \times 1017]150,000 \approx 102,640,000$$

That's a ten followed by 2,640,000 zeroes, which would fill 11 volumes the size of Multiplying it all together for the sake of completeness (Step 1 x Step 2 x Step 3 x Step 4):

Probability of your being born: one in 102,685,000

As a comparison, the approximate number of atoms in the known universe is 1080.

So what's the probability of your being born? It's the probability of 2.5 million people getting together — about the population of San Diego — each to play a game of dice with *trillion-sided dice*. They each roll the dice — and they all come up the exact same number — say, 550,343,279,001.

> **"A miracle is an event so unlikely as to be almost impossible. By that definition, I've just proven that you are a miracle."**
> **Dr. Ali Binazir**

Thanks, Dr Binazir, for the one of my favorite pieces to read. What I take from this is quite simple. It is quite astounding how much time and energy we spend on rubbish, it's astounding how much time we spend in a state of not really appreciating our lives, and certainly not making the most of our good fortune.

Imagine you wake up one day and there is a Ferrari with a bow wrapped around it on your driveway. You have no idea where it came from, who gave you this awesome gift, but all you do know is it's yours to enjoy.

Some people immediately ruin it, put sugar in the gas tank, have to work double shifts at their job just to pay for engine repairs and actually start resenting the horrible misfortune they have to have been given a Ferrari.

Some people immediately put it in the garage, when they drive it, they drive it at 5 miles per hour as safely as possible.

Some people get absorbed in the machine itself. They learn all about the engine, how it works, its capabilities, any upgrades available, and they treat it with respect, but still enjoy driving it and testing its limits!

Guess who I would love you to be a little bit more of:) I think the world needs you and it needs your special skills, that which makes you unique and special, and it's imperative that the world becomes a place where you are able to bring those ideas out.

WIZARDRY AND MAGIC.

I always liked the stories of Wizards and magic powers. I always thought that those times were cool, and of course, who wouldn't want to have a pet dragon! One of the major topics of those days was metallurgy. There must be some way to make copper into gold right. Aluminum into platinum. I think one of the biggest secrets still left in the world is that we actually do have this power. Being able to wave the internal magic wand and change one emotion into something else, is the ultimate display of self-mastery.

Our internal climate is not static. You could be having a pretty average when the phone rings and the person on the other end says, "You have won a thousand bucks" and your mood is sure to brighten.

By the same token you can be having the time of your life when your doctor calls and says "Sorry, we have to amputate" and your mood is going to drop a few notches.

Let's focus on what I call the NET EMOTION.

Some of the greatest minds have incredible NET EMOTION. What is NET EMOTION? Well I am glad you asked! The greats have this remarkable ability to change their emotion. It works like this: When they get upset, they turn it into determination. When the feel scared, they find some bravery and then turn that into determination. When they feel despondent, they turn that into determination.

When they get gutted, floored, whipped, their backsides handed to them on a silver platter, they look for answers and then turn that into determination.

That resultant emotion is always complementary to their dreams. It's a magic wand that turns the copper coins into gold.

The world's top performers have this remarkable ability to change emotions. The really elite ones have the ability to change group emotion.

It's imperative that you learn and understand this skill, because in the ever changing sea of emotion, that's bombarded with distraction, complacency, not knowing if you have done enough or too much, tragedy, etc., you will be well served to have an magic cauldron of emotion that nets you out at the same levels of sincerity, honesty, and hard work regardless. This could end up being one of your most important achievements as a person.

Plan a life where you have to make each situation better, whether you like it or not. It's an ultimate show of gratitude: accept a situation you really don't like, did not create and certainly did not wish for, but make it awesome anyway.

CHAPTER 12: FAILURE.

I t's time to put the concept of failure under the microscope. For too long we have had a relatively poor relationship with failure. I can't count the number of times I have heard people saying, "I don't have time" "It's too big of a risk" "If I don't make it this time, I am done" and a variety of other limiting beliefs and statements that serve no purpose other than to stop the person from seeing something through to the end.

The most important thing to remember is that you are GOING TO FAIL. You have to. You need to. So, stop obsessing over it. You will fail as many times as you need before you get it right. This could be 3 times, 80 times, 500 times or more, and you will never know what that number is until you…. get it right. Capiche?

One of the great joys of this world is seeing some wunderkind who can do what you have been trying to master for 10 years, on his first attempt, but this is life, and deal with it we must.

If there is only one thing we must take from this book, it must be a relentless and merciless attitude towards failure. Failure, my little unwelcome friend, we have a plan for you.

Logically, failure is a crucial part of your learning something. You are always failing, until the magical moment when you succeed, so it really shouldn't be too much of a surprise to fail. What we want is to know how to use those failures to build a

better next attempt. For this, we need to data-mine our failures. And for successful data mining, we need objectivity.

I have a great story about a tournament in India that has become my reference point for failure. My doubles partner and I show up in India as the number 1 seeds for the tournament and are excited to play some good tennis. While checking into the hotel, we notice a well-dressed fellow following us around but not speaking. We come downstairs, rent a Puk-Puk and head to the courts. He jumps in a beat-up Mercedes and follows us. We go to eat, he is there, a small distance away. We go to the gym, he is there. I go for a 5:00 am run, he is there. This goes on for two days, my doubles partner and I starting to get more and more worried that the Indian Mafia has a hit out on us, or we are about to get sold into slavery. We finally go to the tournament director and tell him we think we are being followed. Perhaps it's time to get the five-o, police involved, that sort of a thing. He smiles and says, "Guys, that's your driver for the week." We instantly made friends, and our week turned out way better than it ever could have without him, he showed us some amazing historical spots, taught us about local culture and custom, and took us to places where we could trust the food and dine on delicious local cuisine.

So, it is with failure. Too many of us are in a fear/hate relationship with failure, when we really should be making friends with one of the best tour guides to success that we will ever have.

THE TIME HAS COME TO MASTER THE ART OF FAILING LIKE A CHAMP

- THE HUNTER BECOMES THE HUNTED: Stop hiding from Failure, and instead start seeking it out. It's important to understand that learning is a dynamic process, and it's going to take more than a handful of failures to really master your particular trade. Once you actually develop this understanding, you want to start seeking out failure in areas that you want to improve.

- FAIL OFTEN: If you can make it a habit to put some things onto your rolodex that are challenging and you will most likely fail at a couple of times, then you are on the sure-fire path towards growth.

- FAIL ON PURPOSE: We spend so much of our time trying not to fail, when in reality it should be the other way around. Doing something successfully means you already know how to do it. Doing something and failing means you don't know how to do it.

- GET KNOWLEDGE- because you don't know about certain things until you find out about them. There is no better ingredient to success than applied knowledge. There is almost a 100% chance that inside your failure there is a gap in knowledge, and so with each failure we must be striving to fill in those gaps. You must be chasing new information.

- FAIL FORWARDS: Each failure should be a purposeful attempt at an integration of new information based on the clear evidence presented by your previous attempt. Too often the embarrassment, the anger and the other emotions mean that we fail almost the same way every time, because we are not doing the exercise of planning the modifications. Start looking at your failures with the objective eye and making reasonable, valid modifications, and you will start to fail towards success.

Learn to sit with pain.

When we have something that hurts, our first reaction is to immediately stop the pain. Your body gives you pain when you chop your finger open, because, well, your finger is chopped open and if you don't attend to cleaning it and repairing it, you run the risk of a whole host of infections, problems, and diseases. Pain in this instance therefore serves an incredibly important function.

Emotional pain is an entirely different matter. It enters the realm of the subjective, which means it is different for almost everyone. This means that for some people a certain event is almost intolerable, while with others the same event can be absorbed quite nonchalantly as they carry on with their day. Learning to sit with your pain for a while means not jumping up and acting every time, you have an emotional pain response in your system. Instead knowing that that feeling will be diluted over time and waiting enough for it to have subsided to the point where rational and exact planning can take the place of impulse and pure reaction.

Learning to sit with pain, gives you control over your response, and stops dead in its tracks the process where your emotions, and in this case emotional pain control you.

LEARNED HELPLESSNESS.

A remarkable result of failure can be what has come to be known in clinical terms as learned helplessness. In a famous experiment by Seligman and Maier using dogs, they showed that repeated failure can cause the dogs to eventually not even seek a solution. At first there is an environment where the action taken by the dogs does not solve the problem. The experiment then changes the circumstances to where the initial response would solve the problem, but the dogs simply assumed that they would fail again and refrain from making any attempt.

It is critical to examine whether your own viewpoint or perspective have created this sort of an environment for you. You have been shocked by previous failures and have developed a perspective that you have no control over outcomes and therefore there is no value in trying.

In a healthy internal ecosystem, rather than resisting your problems, we would expect to see full immersion in an attempt to solve them. A person who is not bound by limitations feels as though their current problems actually go a step deeper and are a part of the theme of taking destiny into your own hands.

They believe their careers and lives will be defined by the problems one overcomes, and so moments that are marked by huge problems actually come with massive opportunity. They offer a wonderful chance to create, brainstorm, and use your imagination to find a solution. This difference in mindset creates a world of difference not only in willingness to make an attempt, but also in the diversity of ideas used in these attempts.

SUCCESS THAT LEADS TO FAILURE VERSUS FAILURE THAT LEADS TO SUCCESS.

As contradictory as this may seem, this is actually a very common occurrence. Using developing athletes as an example here, we often hear the story of the wunderkind athlete who was winning everything in their early years, age 12 up to age 16, but then they get surpassed by their peer group and have a hard time dealing with this. It might sound strange that someone who is winning so much, does not really know how to win, but let me explain. Generally, early on in an endeavor we have what we call the 3 ages.

1. The number of years you have been doing your sport.

2. The developmental age of your body. A 12 years old some kids are built like a 16-year-old, and some are built like an 8-year-old.

3. Emotional maturity age. Some 12-year-old kids think like they are 16 and some think like they are 8.

This translates into a huge discrepancy of natural factors. Obviously a 12-year-old with the body of a 16-year-old and emotional maturity of a 16 year old is going to beat up on one that's built and acts like they are 8. But as they progress through the years, Athlete A does not have to work as hard to be competitive, they simply ply their natural advantages. Athlete B has to overcome major deficits to be competitive. Around 16 to 18 years old, the human body developmentally evens out. Suddenly as both athletes start to reach maturity, the natural physical advantage that athlete A has been using to win has neutralized and is quite even with Athlete B. Athlete B, however, has had many more years of competing with a deficit and having to compromise, improvise, problem solve and deal with the emotional setbacks.

There are a number of factors at play here. Because Athlete A was using "winning" as the signal that they were on track, they always felt comfortable that they were developing well. The critical feedback loop of failing and then proactively making decisions on how to perform and train to overcome this failure never developed fully and as such, the critical computing skills on how to solve problems is years behind.

Emotionally, there is developmental territory that has to be hiked to become an elite level performer. Winning all the time does not give your failure and rejection muscles a chance to work out, and as such they atrophy or develop poorly. This leads to incorrect data processing as failure stops becoming a process for improvement, and a necessary part of extremely high skill-set development, and instead takes asylum in the self-image and belief structure.

What follows is generally an emotional breakdown in the face of defeat. Coping mechanisms are triggered in abundance, emotionality rules the decision-making process, and the reality that the skill set is suddenly years behind sinks in. Knowing they have to play catch up over the next several years, the athlete often chooses quitting instead, and as such, many of the world's most talented early performers end up hardly playing their sport or pastime later on.

How does junior athletic development relate to you? We are not that different to the above development story in the sense that many of us stop our development prematurely. We find jobs, we have families, we settle down. But we also don't really have a development plan past a certain age. There is no feedback loop of failure and next input. The most important lesson we can take from this is that we need to have a master plan and grand design for our lives, as well as a keen sense of where the next mile-markers are. We need to carry with us an understanding of how and where we are going to reach for the next rungs on the ladder. Finally, we need to for once and for all break the loop of identifying ourselves by our failures, and simply learn that growth is a scientific process of attempt, feedback, next better attempt. To move forward, we simply need to jump back into this system and start pushing toward our next breakthrough.

FAULT AND RESPONSIBILITY FOR FAILURE

It is human nature to want to find reasons for events. It might be our greatest critical strength. When we fail, we need to find out why, and we need to find a better way. Unfortunately, there is a fine line between a high accountability, clean next attempt and someone looking to avoid responsibility by assigning the fault onto someone else's shoulders.

The great achievers are always sharpening this lens, they are always very wary of assigning blame or trying to minimize their own responsibility. Once you start playing the game of looking for way out of failure, looking to soften the blow, looking to assign responsibility to the weather, the Spirits or your poor dog Shnookums, you are on a slippery slope to EGO-Ville. Your priority has shifted from enjoying the failure to insulating yourself from it, and this normally leads to the ultimate insulation of a poor or nonexistent next attempt. Stay away from the blame game and focus instead on executing a valid improved attempt.

FAILURE IS THE BIRTHPLACE OF REAL OPPORTUNITY.

Most of us don't even wait for the real world to show us we didn't get the opportunity- we decide before we even send out the resume that it won't be successful. So why even try?

I want everyone here to take a second and think about it:

How many really interesting people did you <u>NOT</u> go and talk to?

How many interviews could you have gone on but didn't?

How many really interesting online courses have you seen, but didn't do?

How many things could you have done that you decided for one reason or another not to do?

It's these self-imposed limits that really can be incredibly determinative when it comes to your ultimate destiny. You have to develop that plucky trait where you just keep digging, picking, scraping and hustling until you finally pull together an opportunity: a call back, and interview, an acceptance to your enrollment letter.

Compare MAN A who makes 5 opportunities for himself and takes 4 out of 5, or MAN B who makes 30 and takes 9 of those. MAN A is capitalizing on 80% of his opportunities, while MAN B is only capturing 30% Yet MAN B is actually capturing twice as many opportunities as MAN A. Imagine for a moment what it would feel like if you were in the middle of a train wreck of a day, blowing a pretty cool occasion, but in the back of your mind, you know your process and discipline will make you another opportunity in the coming weeks. With a steady flow of opportunities coming your way, then you can actually afford to relax and have some fun trying to climb your way out of the hole.

You will get to the point where you enjoy the process of making chances for success, and there is an inevitability that some will work out for you. It would be almost impossible to go 0 for 30 in the example above, there are just too many factors to consider. For example, Bob and you are up for promotion, but Bob actually decides to move to Spain, therefore you get the promotion by default. It is almost a mathematical certainty that you are going to convert, some of the time.

And that's the beauty. Consistently creating opportunities for yourself is going to lead to much less pressure to perform, while internally you are freed up, confident that if one of these does not come through, you will have another one around the corner.

RED-LINING ONE AREA OF YOUR LIFE (TEMPORARILY)

A balanced life is a thing of beauty. It can also be a unicorn. Hard to find and even harder to capture. Generally, pushing for achievement in one of your life's major departments, whether that be health, finances, personal development or any other, will mean that one or two other departments will have to take a backseat, and so begins a delicate dance with your life category limits.

Let's say for example you have decided to dedicate yourself to finishing your PHD. The new allotment of time to this cause will mean you need to cut back on socializing and cut back on sleep. You might find you trigger some new coping mechanisms, put on a few pounds and lose a few friends as you move the boundary lines of your health and social life in order to fit in your new goal, the PHD

For the most part, any one of the big life categories above can tolerate being temporarily off balance, as long as there is a deliberate plan to move those boundary lines back as soon as is humanly possible.

In a perfect world, this would not need to be the case, as you could simply switch from one idea to the next, but in the real world, start-ups, PHD's, extra community projects and the like are all done in spare time, carved out of already full schedules.

The bottom line here is you need to be mentally prepared to have a report card that brings you some b's and c's in some categories for a semester or two, while you shoot for the stars in one major new goal.

FAILURE TO SEE RESULTS. CHANGE. IT'S HAPPENING, TRUST ME.

Change is an extremely funny thing. Change can be delicate and subtle. Take the emergence of Netflix. The folks at Blockbuster could not possibly have known that they were doomed. The market didn't know either, but the reality was, in fact, that Netflix had ushered in a whole new era. The same was true when television replaced radio. Radio stars were huge, and most people would never have guessed that their favorite stars would soon be obsolete. The same is true when you are building a new you. The internal currents that create lasting change are hard at work behind the scenes. Sometimes you don't feel like the work you are putting in is making a difference at all, until that moment you look back and realize that life has changed tremendously.

You will not be where you are now in 10 years' time. There is no doubt about that. You will have undergone significant change. As far as pure goal stopping power, there is nothing that derails us more than simply not seeing the results when we want them and then deciding that they are actually not coming. This is what leads us to stop and give up on ourselves. No amount of failure has the same ultimate stopping power as the individual quitting on themselves.

You have to continue your process. Bolster that belief inside a realistic framework.

Life has this funny way of surprising to the upside! You know, I see so many people who are saddened, and stuck and not achieving the results they want, but yet these people are also the people who do the most forecasting of the future. So, you don't know who you are going to bump into, you don't know who is going to be impressed by your polished look, your sense of humor, your "insert skill here" that you have been working on. You don't know what opportunity is right around the corner, you don't know what the needs of the marketplace are and when those needs will coincide with your skill set.

Failure is the friend you never knew you had. He is a wealth of very relevant information. He is consistent in giving you insights into how you can improve and do better next time. Go up to him and give him a hug, shake hands and make friends. You just took on a new team member. Destiny just got goosebumps, he knows you are coming to pay him a visit next.

Chapter 13: Turning the Lens Toward Humanity

The earth is a dynamic living planet, and our part on it must surely be to nurture and look after her. Humans as a species have left quite the mark on our host. You can see our lights from outer space. You can see physical structures we have built from outer space. There are 7 billion of us and counting, all using this little lonely planet as the stage to play out our lives, our dreams and our ambitions as the story of us unfolds.

We all carry with us a great responsibility. We should be focusing our resources and skillsets on building a sustainable, healthy planet. We should all be keenly aware of the part that we must play in achieving this goal.

It's easy to paint a picture of us as the great custodians of our planet. Walking hand in hand with the plant species, animal populations on the rise in conjunction with an ever-shrinking endangered species list. Our engineering, farming and development perfectly tuned to maintaining a balance between the needs mankind and maintaining the health of our planet. It feels good to imagine humans as the masters of applied knowledge.

I believe we have arrived at a critical point for mankind, where for each and every one of us, we must add one more segment into our master goals list. goals list. Right now, the list is comprised mainly of the big six,

Health, Family, Personal Development, Finances, Social Life, and Career, but I believe there should be a new entrant:

My part in looking after planet.

Mental health and toughness of the people is a critical first step. Wars, destruction, and violence toward one another, plants and animals, as well as our precious eco systems is not a sustainable model. Building ourselves to be driven by bigger ideas than ego and money, and to be ready to be a high-level contributor to both our communities and the environment is a natural next evolutionary step. Relying on big corporations to do the right thing is as dangerous as it is unlikely, and as such we need to point our technology towards accountability and monitoring the health of the systems we rely on for survival.

Building an intelligent, iron mind, will free you up to reach down and help others by transferring your strength. It will also free you up to use your precious time to stay educated and focused on the long term greater good.

HOW IS MOTHER EARTH DOING?

Right now, we have some pretty awesome challenges facing us. We are in a race to beat climate change, and this means getting to zero emissions in a number of economic categories.

We are all well versed in the progress we have made with generating power. We have wind farms going up, we have massive solar installations. We have companies like Tesla and a host of competitors coming on the market soon. We have companies like Uber tackling the need for ownership, and possibly driving down the resource hungry nature of ownership.

Keep in mind that the picture is bigger than this, as we also have to account for the ecological footprint and emissions of Agriculture, Transportation, and manufacturing as they make up a formidable part of the greenhouse gas emissions in each economy.

Not only are we in a race to get the emissions of these sectors down to zero, we are also in a race to scale them up to meet the coming demands of a growing population on earth.

The current estimates are that the number of buildings on earth will double over the next 40 years. Think about how much steel, concrete, wood, and other natural resources that is. Our economic models need to make a late-in-the-game change to reflect not only the profits and potential economic windfalls of this gigantic coming growth, but also to have a more exact accounting for the actual cost in terms of help or damage to the eco systems and health of the planet. We will need a much better system of monitoring all of this information, so that it does not slip into the background of business as usual as critical ecosystems collapse and irreparable damage is done to the planet.

It's going to be imperative that we see a shift in what the media is reporting, so that we are all far more in tune and informed as to the health and progress of efforts to solve effectively the problem of managed human growth in conjunction with managed ecological solutions.

We all know what the DOW Jones Industrial average is. We all know that there is a number that it spits out, 25,800 as of this writing that attests to the health of the companies that make up the index.

I would love to see a similar ecological number. Wake up in the morning and see the USA Ecological average at 20,000. A sector by sector breakdown would show improvements in various sectors, and where we have lost ground. We, the public would be much more informed, and would have a way of holding ourselves and the people who represent us in government accountable for making continued progress. Tennis has just adopted something similar called the Universal Tennis Rating, which is an algorithm driven ranking system that considers various factors in each tennis playing country and spits out a remarkably accurate number for how good a tennis player is on a global scale. The technology and math are available and we could achieve this. With a swipe of your finger, you can check your heartbeat on your iPhone, and with just one more swipe, you could monitor the health of the planet. Pretty cool.

It would be nice to see potential candidates campaigning on their ecological plans and promising to divert money away from building aircraft carriers and weapons that have only the potential to create destruction, but instead budgets for ecological solutions being the order of the day. If we repurposed just 10% of the budgets we have set aside for military use, I'll bet we could make monumental progress.

BRAND NEW ECO ARCHITECTURE

The very limit of technology has been tested by some of the most awesome projects on earth. Anyone who has travelled to Dubai will attest to the spectacle that is the Burj Khalifa, the world's tallest building. Then there is the monumental scale and achievement is architecture and engineering that is the Palm Islands.

What about the Cayan Tower, the world's second tallest building. It's hard to describe the level of "Let's take this baby all the way to the limit" that was going through the minds of its developers. Not only does it rotate 90 degrees from base to roof, but it also is a world first having no structural pillars.

Next step I believe is going to be monumental eco-building achievements. Pushing the limits of design to create buildings that capture and store enormous amounts of energy, have zero emissions, and contain produce and plant life as part of the design.

Imagine if each city center had one high rise building dedicated to farming, Hi-Rise Hydroponic farming. The demands for water, the footprint of transporting the produce would be dropped to near zero. An amazon drone could bring it to your doorstep in minutes.

MASSIVE MULTI COUNTRY PARTNERSHIPS

The large hadron collider is not only remarkable for being the biggest and most complex machine ever built, it was also a landmark partnership between 22, member states. The European Organization for Nuclear research, better known as CERN (Conseil Europeen pour la recherche Nucleaire) spent about 13.25 billion to hunt down the Higgs boson!

I imagine similar partnerships raising funds and spending whatever is necessary to facilitate the necessary ecological breakthroughs from state-of-the-art Eco research labs, and funding the eco-entrepreneurs of tomorrow.

TRANSCENDING THE WALLS OF THE CLASSROOM.

We have made enormous progress in dealing with poverty. In fact, the number of people worldwide living on less than two dollars per day has fallen from 36% to right around 10% over the last 30 years, a truly remarkable achievement.

Unfortunately, Africa has not had the same success, and has actually seen an increase of people living in extreme poverty. As you might imagine, it becomes extremely difficult to build and mobilize your economy if you have vast numbers of uneducated people living in poverty. They will not be demanding high paying jobs that produce revenue for the government in the form of taxes, which then can be used to build out infrastructure and grow the economy. That loop is severely impacted by lack of education, and thus it becomes imperative that we form global initiatives to continue the fantastic progress made over the last 30 years, and of course, bring Sub Saharan Africa squarely into the picture.

Uneducated populations need to become a thing of the past. Just as Uber has made it possible for the redundancies that were your extra 3 seats in your car to be put back into useful circulation, there should be a similar breakthrough in education soon. The technology is there. And for all the dictators who hate this idea, maybe your path to being mentally tough could remember that 1% of a trillion is a lot more than 1% of a billion. Empowering and helping your populations grow actually makes sense, even from a corrupt Dictators point of view :)

THE FIRST PLASTICS BILLIONAIRE

We have an enormous amount of spare plastic. Right now, it's floating around in our oceans and getting put into landfills. But what if we cracked the plastic code.

There must be a way to turn those plastics back into a fuel of some kind, so instead of using oil, we could consume our plastic supplies in the form of energy instead. Someone, somewhere with the know how should be hard at work on solving this problem.

We could also build with Plastic. There is a company in Africa doing this already, filling used bottles with sand and then cementing them together to make shelters. Considering the enormous amounts of people needing shelter, and the enormous amounts of bottles killing fish by the gazillion, it makes sense to repurpose that waste into habitats for people who would otherwise be pretty much sleeping in a shack.

In conclusion, humanity is moving swiftly towards its future. A future that seems brighter than ever, and our ever-creating genius is capable of solving the most ardent and pressing of problems. Turning ourselves into a mentally tough species means facing these challenges head on, and using our toughness to make the right choices, regardless of impulse and past habit.

Change is indeed afoot, and we are excited to chase it in a mentally tough way.

Thanks to everyone for spending this time with me, I wish you an incredible journey, one that is laden with success of every kind, and that paves the way for future generations with a beautiful, clean and highly functioning planet.

32897184R00134

Made in the USA
San Bernardino, CA
17 April 2019